KEYS TO WINNING PHYSICIAN SUPPORT

Second Edition

Real winners don't gag the good guys

By Richard E. Thompson, MD

American College of Physician Executives
Suite 200
4890 West Kennedy Boulevard
Tampa, Florida 33609
813/287-8000

ISBN: 0-924674-68-7
Library of Congress Card Number: 98-88204

Printed in the United States of America by Hillsboro Printing Company, Tampa, Florida.

Current Wisdom

The average medical man is an educated gentleman, a delightful companion, a man of parts, and many such are our best friends. But doctors, when associated in corporate matters, are oftentimes too self-seeking. With an eye out for their profession, they are inclined to be aggressive, and naturally, under such conditions are not a gracious, peaceful, easily cooperative body of men.

This professional enthusiasm is apt to obscure an all-around view of hospital government.—George H.M. Rowe, M.D., Association of Hospital Superintendents, 1902.

Interdependence is a higher value than independence.—Stephen S. Covey, *The Seven Habits of Highly Effective People: Powerful Lessons in Personal Change.* New York, N.Y.: Fireside Books, 1989, p. 9.

Foreword

It would be comforting to say that much has changed since this book was first published back in 1991. Take comfort, then, for much has changed. Health care is increasingly dominated by managed care organizations and operations, and the overall system is integrating at a dizzying pace. But, to a large extent, the changes have been in magnitude and direction. The underlying actors and forces that have shaped the health care delivery and financing system over the past decade are much the same. Even though the role of managed care has intensified, and the elements of the system are constantly shifting and rearranging themselves to accommodate pressures from payers and policy makers, health care is still delivered by clinicians, mostly traditional doctors, and the purpose of the system, in spite of an increasing emphasis on the business of health, is to maintain and improve the health of our citizens.

It remains Dr. Thompson's contention in this new edition of his book that the adversarial relationship that frequently exists and even more frequently threatens to erupt between physicians and their nonphysician colleagues serves no one well. His is both a call for cooperation and a roadmap to its achievement. The message is greatly augmented by Dr. Thompson's wry sense of humor and by his clear belief that the system can be made to work before it has become thoroughly broken. We are led to believe that it is Dr. Thompson's style and commitment that made the first edition of this book one of our best sellers. Those commodities continue to define this project. This is a good "read." It is also good advice. Everyone's goals will be better served if the route is approached with a smile rather than a dagger. I can only hope you enjoy reading the book as much as I enjoyed editing it.

Wesley Curry
Managing Editor
Book Publishing
American College of Physician Executives
November 1998

About the Author

Richard E. Thompson, MD received his bachelor's degree from Vanderbilt University, Nashville, Tennessee, in 1955, and his medical degree from Washington University Medical School, St. Louis, Missouri (cum laude, AOA, 1959). He is the author of more than 100 articles and books, including *Health Care Reform as Social Change*, ACPE, Tampa,1993; *So You've Been Integrated, Now What: Opportunities for Physicians Practicing in Managed Care Settings*, ACPE, Tampa, 1996; *The Medical Staff Leader's Practical Guide*, 3rd Edition, Opus, Marblehead, Massachusetts, 1996; and "Sustainability as the Linchpin of Public Policy and Industry Initiatives," *Physician Executive*, July/August 1998, page 52.

Once a practicing pediatrician (Denver area, 1964-70); Chief of Pediatrics and neonatologist at the Columbus (Georgia) Medical Center and simultaneously Assistant Professor of Pediatrics at Emory University, Atlanta, Georgia (1970-74); Deputy Director of JCAHO's Quality Resource Center (1974-75); and a Vice President of the Illinois Hospital Association (1975-79), Dr. Thompson has free-lanced as an author, public speaker, and consultant since 1979 at Thompson, Mohr and Associates, Inc. (P.O. Box 1497, Dunedin, FL, 34697). Dr. Thompson's e-mail address is richthom@aol.com.

Dr. Thompson is creator of the humor book, *Things You'll Learn If You Live Long Enough*, Celex/Great Quotations, Lombard, Illinois (1990 and 1996), and a columnist for the Bolivar Missouri *Herald and Free Press*. His main hobby is publishing and distributing (free) a monthly humor and commentary letter, *Between the Lines*.

How to Get True Value out of This Book

- *Read* this book. Or at least scan the "boxes" containing key points that are scattered throughout this book. *Discuss* points that interest you with other members of the leadership team (including physician leaders) individually and in meetings.

- *Distribute* copies of the book to co-workers, both management staff and physicians.

- *Use* the book, including the Points for Discussion at the end of each chapter and Cases for Discussion in the Appendix, as a resource at retreats and as a basis for making educational presentations to both management staff and physicians.

- *Refer* to this book for useful reminders when dealing with issues involving physician leaders and practicing clinicians.

For best results, also read and discuss this book's companion volume, *So You've Been Integrated, Now What: Opportunities for Physicians Practicing in Managed Care Settings*, ACPE, 1996.

Note: This book should be a great help to executives and managers who have no clinical background and/or who have little experience dealing with doctors. But it also should prove useful to physician executives and physician leaders (see Glossary for definition of physician leader). That's because even MD and DO executives, managers, and clinician-leaders must cultivate special skills to work effectively with practicing clinicians in an organizational context.

Glossary

Life is too short for two people to argue when they don't really disagree.
The key to avoiding misunderstandings is careful definition of terms.

The following definitions are contextual, meaning this is how these words and phrases are used in this book.

Administration is used in the neutral, dictionary sense of "one who administers something." Executives and managers care for administrative details, and so do physician leaders.

Clinical Expertise means a body of knowledge and skills dealing with the anatomy and the physiology of the human body and with diagnosis and treatment of illness and injury.

The clinical expertise of each physician is a unique product of the individual's selection of specialty or subspecialty, the degree to which the individual currently engages in clinical practice, and relevant continuing medical education.

Clinical Practice does not mean "private practice" or any other practice arrangement. It means the difficult task of modifying practice guidelines to fit the unique needs of each individual who receives health care services.

Therefore, examples of "practicing physicians" include a hospital-based anesthesiologist, an internist in "private practice," a general surgeon employed by or contracting with a managed care organization, a family physician in a large multispecialty clinic, and a skilled subspecialist on the faculty of a medical university.

Clinical Practice Guidelines differ from Clinical Pathways in that they specifically relate to the decision-making process of the practitioner primarily responsible (and liable) for an individual's medical care. That is usually an MD or a DO. This practicing physician is the CEO in the context of caring for individual patients.

Clinical Pathways are step-by-step roadmaps. A critical pathway includes activities of all clinical professionals (practicing physicians, nurses, clinical technicians) on whom a specific patient, resident, or client depends for medical care.

Data and Information. A data system is simply a source of raw, uninterpreted statistics. Information is the set of conclusions drawn from data and daily observations by responsible individuals.

"DO" means an individual who has earned the postgraduate doctor of osteopathy degree.

Executive means a person whose training is primarily in business, finance, managing data and people, and establishing organizational systems. The owners, through a governing body, give the chief executive the responsibility and limited authority to carry out (execute) principles, policies, goals, plans, and objectives of the organization.

Executive Function. The executive function in organizations means that an individual or group is authorized to execute, or carry out, on a day-to-day basis, the policies of the organization and is entrusted with the responsibility to act on a daily basis to direct the organization's activities.

Health Care is a term of recent origin, used by politicians, insurance companies, and managers of provider organizations to encompass both "wellness" services and medical care.

Health Care Executive means an executive in a health care organization.

Health Care Manager means an individual who provides needed organizational support to physicians, nurses, clinical technicians, and others who interact on the front line with those receiving health care services.

IDS means integrated delivery system. The term IDS is not synonymous with managed care organization and does not imply any specific funding mechanism. An IDS is simply an integrated network of health care professionals and supporting managers that provides a convenient and efficient opportunity for people in need of any health care service to receive it from the same provider. An IDS is true reality—that is, an entity that can be visited. (For contrast, see the definition of managed care organization.)

Managed Care is sometimes used to refer to the current U.S. health care policy of "managed competition," unique in the world because the primary goal is maximizing investor profit. Managed Care is also used to mean management of the individual patient (or client, or resident, whatever is applicable in the various components of the IDS) by clinical practitioners who modify clinical practice guidelines and clinical pathways to fit the unique needs of members and beneficiaries who are users of medical care services offered by the IDS.

Managed Care Organization (MCO) means an entity that exists only on paper. An MCO is virtual reality, as opposed to the true reality of an IDS. The purpose of an MCO is to take advantage of current national and state health care policy that encourages profit-taking and purports to allow market forces to control costs and ensure dependability of medical services.

Managed Competition refers to current U.S. health care policy. Competition is "managed" by a complex set of federal and state laws and regulations.

"MD" means an individual who has earned the postgraduate doctor of medicine degree.

Medical Care Services means health care services provided because an individual is ill or injured.

Medical Executive Committee (MEC). The representatives of the medical staff authorized to accomplish the medical executive function, in concert with the medical staff president and the vice president for medical affairs (VPMA).

Physician means an MD or DO whose primary activity is providing the physician component of medical care services. See also clinical practice.

It is important to note that all physicians are MDs or DOs, but not all MDs and DOs are physicians. For example, an executive who claims to have included "physician input" in the decision-making process but who has input only from MDs or DOs who are not frontline practicing physicians is, however inadvertently, making a mistake that could prove costly.

Physician Executive means an individual who, in whatever sequence, has acquired both clinical expertise and executive expertise and whose primary activities as an executive include interacting with both physicians and executives.

Physician Leader, in the context of this book, means an MD or DO who chooses to remain primarily a frontline clinical practitioner but who also accepts a responsible position of organizational leadership. Examples include clinical department chairs/directors, the president of the medical staff in the old-model "organized medical staff" in hospitals, members of a health care system's medical advisory group (MAG), etc.

Quality in the context of this book means dependable performance from the viewpoint of users of health care services provided by an IDS.

Shared Leadership in the context of this book means a seat at the table when the final decision is made and the authority to help create implementation strategies.

Table of Contents

From "Physician Input" to Empowerment and Shared Leadership

> *Why the change from physician input to shared leadership?*

Physicians. Bah Humbug! Who Needs 'Em?

> *Follow the money.*
> *Isn't "shared power" an oxymoron?*
> *There is an alternative: no physicians.*
> *Shared power is the reality of health care.*
> *The value equation must be balanced.*
> *One aspect of compliance: JCAHO accreditation.*
> *When only a doctor will do.*
> *Physicians are important at all organizational levels.*
> *The executive edge.*

Why Shared Leadership Is Difficult. Part 1: I Didn't Even Know He Sold His House

> *The added value of different perspectives.*
> *Is your goal short-term or long-range?*

Why Sharing Leadership Is Difficult. Part 2: Fifty-Fifty, like Rabbit Fajitas

> *Bet I can hold a grudge longer than you can.*
> *The rabbit fajitas joint venture.*
> *The phone poll with still-relevant results.*
> *The impact of recent events.*

Why Sharing Leadership Is Difficult. Part 3: Who's in Charge

> *Creating an annual budget for the organization.*
> *Preparing and safeguarding the medical records of patients,*
> *clients, and residents.*
> *Credentialing and privileging independent practitioners.*
> *The ultimate example of needing careful clarification of responsibilities: Clinical*
> *care of each individual patient, client, or resident.*

Introduction

Working with physicians is a unique challenge that has been likened to petting a bumblebee[1] or driving a nitroglycerin truck.[2]

This book is not about "partnering" in the economic or legal sense of the word. Rather, this book is meant to help executives, managers, practicing physicians, and physician leaders appreciate one another's skills and value, so that they can effectively share leadership and thus all achieve success.

The reader will quickly discover that this book goes way beyond old and obsolete practices such as playing golf with the "heavy admitters," referring to "the doctor's workshop," and bribing doctors to be "loyal." The book also shies away from potential pitfalls inherent in Machiavellian manipulation of doctors.

Everybody knows how to throw money at doctors. This book gives you an extra edge, so that sought-after physicians will choose to partner with you rather than with your competition.

Physicians remain in the top 5 percent of the population in terms of income. That partly explains why throwing money at doctors does not guarantee a good working relationship. Besides, doctors want more from you than money. For example, many physicians truly want to participate in decisions that will, over time, either preserve or destroy professionalism in the evolving managed care health system (or in whatever model follows if it turns out that professionalism cannot be maintained by any means in an investor-profit health care model).[3,4]

References

1. Grayson, M. "How to Pet a Bumblebee." *Hospitals and Health Networks* 70(3):7, Feb. 5, 1996.

2. Goldsmith, J. "Building Integrated Systems—Driving the Nitroglycerin Truck." *Healthcare Forum Journal* 36(2):36-8,40,44, March-April, 1993.

3. Kassirer, J. "Managing Care: Should We Adopt a New Ethic?" *New England Journal of Medicine* 339(6):397-8, Aug. 6, 1998.

4. Shortell, S., and others. "Physicians as Double Agents. Maintaining Trust in an Era of Multiple Accountabillities." *JAMA* 280(12):1102-8, Sept.23-30, 1998.

Chapter 1

From "Physician Input" to
Empowerment and Shared Leadership

Shared Leadership *in the context of this book means a seat at the table when the final decision is made and the authority to help create implementation strategies.*

In today's health care system, successful executives and physicians are those who truly empower one another and practice shared leadership.

When the first edition of this book was written in 1991, we were nearing the end of the separatist era in U.S. health care. In that era, health care entities, such as hospitals, solo physician office practices, and single-specialty group practices, were all independently organized. And relationships between these independent entities were usually stormy.

Retreats and seminars on "hospital/medical staff relations" and "physician/executive conflict" abounded. Everyone understood that, when a medical executive committee met in "executive session," the term was a euphemism for dis-inviting the "administrator" or CEO. "Should physicians be on the board?" was a question often raised by physicians complaining that board mistakes were made because of not enough "physician input." In some cases, however, this complaint reflected an unreasonable expectation that the CEO and the board should consult every physician on the staff before making important decisions. High CEO turnover rates were attributed partly to effective physician efforts to get boards to "fire administrators." At the same time, executives of that era may someday admit that they used medical staff bylaws as a tool to manipulate, control, and even get rid of some "medical staff members." Overall, executives and board members on one hand, and a variety of powerful physician factions on the other, did not trust each other with their secret plans, which everybody knew all about anyway.

Unfortunately, that tense and negative dynamic is not yet ancient history. In fact, the degree to which it is still operative in some locations is quite surprising. But, thank goodness, the tension isn't the norm anymore. In spite of the eagerness of today's aggressive investigative press to paint a contrary image, the picture of executives stuffing gags in the mouths of their physicians is not accurate in many managed care settings.

Value-added management, with (carefully defined) shared leadership between executives, frontline clinicians, and individual physician leaders, is on the horizon. Just in time.

Why the Change from Physician Input to Shared Leadership?

It's tempting to wax eloquent and talk about "new paradigms" and "new millennium management." But, frankly, the positive turn in the working relationship between (most) executives and (most) physicians has little to do with the coming of a new millennium. Rather, the evolution of genuine shared leadership is coming about because:

- Executives and managers finally realize that they cannot deliver the health care services promised by the organization, even by employing or contracting with an army of consultants, attorneys, and data processing specialists. To paraphrase a buzzphrase of recent years: "No Medicine, No Margin."

- Simultaneously, most physicians have come to admit that practicing physicians are ill-prepared to manage the complexities of today's politically controlled insurance and Medicare systems, which are, ironically, characterized by detailed regulations that control the managed care "free market." Plus, operational details such as human resources issues and budgeting have never been major strong points of practicing physicians. In other words: "No Management, No Margin either!"

- The advantages of practicing in a well-managed organization with a salary or contract arrangement, as opposed to freelancing as a "private practitioner," are now well-recognized by many physicians. With each passing year, physicians young and old are less likely to mourn the loss of an "autonomy" that was never as complete as some imagined and that had drawbacks at least equal to its advantages. At least that was my experience in "private pediatric practice" (see figure on page 3).

- As part of the evolving relationship, individuals trained in business management now want to know more about the true nature of medical practice responsibility. Practice "guidelines" are increasingly appreciated as guidelines. The realization is sinking in that use of clinical guidelines will not eliminate individual clinical decision making (the source of a physician's power) in health care.

- The macho management style tried by some who attempted to treat physicians like assembly-line laborers did not work well, either in terms of retaining truly sought-after physicians or in terms of a positive public image that is so necessary to marketing success. So some executive groups, like soccer teams, seem ready to back off a little, regroup, and take another path toward the goal.

The Myth and the Reality of Presumed "Physician Autonomy" in the "Good Old Days"

I am my own boss; my time is my own.

The private practice physician was at the beck and call of each family for whom he or she assumed responsibility and did not relinquish this responsibility even when he or she delegated an "on-call" physician to cover his or her practice. In addition, sought-after physicians might be called at any time to provide a clinical consultation for a colleague. The private practicing physician was never really his or her own boss.

I am licensed as a physician and therefore can do anything I want in clinical practice. That is, my license authorizes me to do "the skin and its contents."

The language of state licensure acts still implies such broad permission. But, actually, limitations on practice patterns have always been imposed, at first by hospital rules and peer review, then for more than 20 years now by granting only those "individual-specific clinical privileges" that match an individual's postgraduate training and experience.

I can work in any hospital I want to.

The author finished one year of pediatric residency at Denver Children's Hospital (DCH), then entered "general practice." Requests for privileges at Denver Children's Hospital were denied until after the author had completed a residency at DCH, includinf serving as chief resident.

I can make more money in "private practice."

For some, that may be true. But the doctor kept less of the money he or she made in those days. The doctor in "private practice" spent money on business expenses; employee perks; duplicating equipment in doctors' offices; and buying, building, or renting buildings.

I can give better quality patient care if I'm in autonomous "private practice."

Nonsense. Resources available to patients and the convenience of accessing them are definitely superior in ethically run, integrated health care delivery system than when "private practice" offices, laboratories, rehabilitation services, etc. were scattered all over town.

The physician-patient relationship was better when the patient viewed me as being autonomous.

Not necessarily, The physician-patient relationship is whatever the physician chooses to make it, regardless of organizational efforts to control that relationship.

- Compared to a few years ago, more physicians today are better prepared to be part of organizational management. Many physicians who remain primarily clinicians have developed a good understanding of how organizations work and have developed good organizational skills, such as analytical and communication skills.

- Once, "physician leader" was an oxymoron except in the arena of medical society politics. That is no longer true. And a larger number of frontline clinicians who do not choose to be part of leadership have become quite savvy about working as part of an organization.[1]

- Management principles embraced by many since 1990, such as "drive out fear" and "empowerment" of co-workers, are now recognized as useful techniques for establishing and maintaining a good executive/physician working relationship.

By the way, kudos to pioneer physician executives of a few short years ago. These first-in-the-field workers chose to develop a valuable blend of clinical and executive skills, bridged a once-wide abyss between clinicians and business-trained executives, and thus contributed greatly to the emergence and evolution of true shared leadership in health care organizations.

Discussion Points

1. In your organization, what are some examples of "shared leadership?" In these examples, do executives and physicians truly empower each other?

2. In your organization, are there any barriers to sharing leadership? If so, what are they?

3. How can barriers to sharing leadership be overcome? Be specific. What is step 1, and who should take it?

4. The Joint Commission on Accreditation of Healthcare Organizations (JCAHO) requires, in the hospital component of the integrated delivery system, "a mechanism designed to provide effective communication among the medical staff, administration, and governing body."[2] In your organization, how is this requirement met?

   Would this be a good idea even if JCAHO did not require it? If so, why? If not, why not?

5. JCAHO requires that, "If there are multiple levels of governance, there is an established mechanism for the medical staff to communicate with *all levels* [emphasis added] of governance involved in policy decisions affecting patient care services at the hospital."[3]

   In your organization, how is this requirement met?

   Would this be a good idea even if JCAHO did not require it? If so, why? If not, why not?

6. In the early days of "managed care," some health care and insurance company executives made the mistake of trying to "gag" physicians, meaning prevent (not discourage; prevent, as in forbid) physicians from telling patients if they needed costly medical services.

    Was this a good idea? Why or why not? Could managed care have achieved reduced costs without this early tactic? Would this have occurred in a managed care organization in which executives shared leadership with responsible physicians? Why or why not?

References

1. Thompson, R. "How to Exercise Power When You Have Limited Authority." *Family Practice Management* 5(1):82-4, Jan. 1998.

2. *1998 Hospital Accreditation Standards* ("pocket-size" edition). Oakbrook Terrace, Ill.: Joint Commission on Accreditation of Healthcare Organizations, MS.2.3.6, page 227.

3. *Ibid.*, MS.2.3.6.1, page 227.

Chapter 2
Physicians! Bah Humbug! Who Needs 'Em?

Follow the Money

So far, only one certainty has emerged from the discordant cacophony that was the Great Health Care Reform Debate of 1993-94.

Health care dollars will never again flow easily to separatists.[1]

The economic reality is that physicians and health care executives must now empower each other and practice genuinely shared leadership if either group is to succeed.

Isn't "Shared Power" an Oxymoron?

"Shared power" is only an oxymoron if your management style is similar to that of Chainsaw Al. Sure, executives with a dictatorial management style abhor the very notion of sharing leadership. In fact, even executives who do not have a dictatorial style must often feel frustrated by the need to coax, cajole, persuade, and explain. Every busy executive must occasionally wonder in secret if time spent sharing the decision-making process is really productive time. After all, when one has all the answers, one is usually eager to act.

But take a careful look at the style of executives with great staying power. Most of them appreciate that achieving "buy-in" to goals and plans is necessary if success is to be achieved.

One main lesson of the CQI (continuous quality improvement) era is that empowering and listening to co-workers, even to the point of giving in on an issue now and then, enhances job satisfaction and hence increases productivity. Especially when physicians are part of an organizational mix, an executive who chooses to flaunt authority and attempts to force compliance with his or her wishes may someday find him- or herself outmaneuvered, and without enough support to function effectively. But an executive who downplays authority and instead controls with effective persuasion and open, honest communication can ordinarily expect a loyal following, a profitable bottom line, and enviable high-level job security.

There Is an Alternative: No Physicians

If you can figure out how to run a successful health care entity without any physicians at all, your life will be greatly simplified. In addition, you will make millions overnight by selling your secret!

But until that day, the best strategy is to be aware of some reasons that, consciously or unconsciously, you depend on frontline clinicians and physician leaders. Here are a few examples.

Shared Power Is the Reality of Health Care

Physicians have power of a type that does not require holding a position of high authority on the organizational chart.

The physician's power results from mastery of unique clinical knowledge and skills, and from the willingness to take a unique kind of responsibility. That is, while the executive may focus on providing revenue-producing wellness services and on marketing to young and healthy plan members, the physician's day is made up of visit after visit with people who are not themselves. The medical doctor is the person who knows what to do and how to do it when enjoyment of life is threatened by poor health. And on the scariest days of people's lives, meaning sudden onset of illness or injury, the doctor is the person who must remain a rock of calmness and objectivity in a sea of concern if not a maelstrom of outright panic. In true medical or surgical emergencies, it is the doctor, not a hospital vice president, who must confidently make quick decisions in the face of incomplete data, given a sense of urgency that does not allow time to gather and ponder more information.

Please don't misunderstand this point. It isn't necessary for the management team to accept the old notion that their work is somehow subservient to a practitioner's every whim. And it is unwise to tolerate arrogant physicians who say, "You can tell me what to do when you go to medical school and get your license to practice medicine!" But it is necessary for those who choose a career in health care management to realize that the reality of their days is sharing leadership with physicians. Confirmation of this reality is fairly easy to find if one chooses to look for it.

For example, in hospitals, where integrated networks take the most economic and legal risks, a fixture in each patient's medical record is the "order sheet." At this writing (rightly or wrongly), it remains true that only doctors can write on the order sheet in most medical records, manual or electronic.

One practical result, as many executives have discovered, is that efforts to improve some target system can be quite disappointing if the system is one put in motion by physicians' orders, yet management does not consider it necessary to involve relevant physicians in efforts to improve that system.

Another practical result of this reality is that financial projections relied upon by the board can miss the mark completely if knowledgeable physicians are not allowed the opportunity to participate in the development of those projections. I was once on the board of a system that opened up new women's and children's medical services. Drawing on my experience as medical director of a neonatology unit, I warned the board to expect initial profits to be far below those projected, because actual costs of providing newborn intensive care had been grossly underestimated. The CEO found this assistance quite helpful.

The Value Equation Must Be Balanced
VALUE = Dependable Services + Reasonable Cost

Today, purchasers of health care services want to award contracts on the basis of overall value, rather than just signing up with the cheapest system.[2-4] Knowledgeable executives are not surprised by this development. After all, CQI principle #4 of Dr. W. Edwards Deming is "End the practice of awarding business on the basis of price alone."[5]

Imagine that tomorrow your organization is expecting a visit from the top brass of a local industry that will soon let a lucrative contract to either you or a competitor. The visiting team includes the company's medical director, who will (among other things) evaluate the priority given to dependable performance in your clinical care settings. Now imagine that (for whatever improbable reason) all of your executives, middle managers, accountants, consultants, attorneys, and lobbyists can make it to work, but none of your physicians, nurses, or clinical technicians can.

Given those unlikely circumstances, what chance would you have of impressing the big brass with efficient financial performance? Presumably a very good chance indeed, either because you really are efficient or because the people needed to create the illusion of efficiency were able to make it to work. But what chance do you have of demonstrating substantively that providing dependable clinical services is as important to you as financial success? The answer is, no chance at all.

Demonstrating a truly balanced value equation, meaning that dependable performance from the viewpoint of users of health care services is as important as profit, is impossible unless practicing physicians and physician leaders are considered as important as other executives and financial consultants.

One Aspect of Compliance: JCAHO Accreditation

Especially in the hospital/medical center component of your integrated system, physician leadership is now critical to avoiding hassles with JCAHO. The Joint Commission once settled for the *illusion* of physician leadership. That is, nonphysicians, such as the Medical Staff Office Coordinator, could satisfy JCAHO by just creating documents and getting physicians to sign them. No more. Today, the executive and management staff cannot achieve and retain JCAHO accreditation without showing JCAHO surveyors *substantive results* of genuine physician leadership. This pertains primarily to patient protective "quality" functions such as credentialing, privileging, and providing data confirming dependable clinician performance.

I don't want the reader to get off track by lapsing into the old, narrow, fearful "the Joint Commission is coming" mode. I want the reader to focus on the positive new opportunities for shared leadership. However, a listing of reasons you need physician leaders would be incomplete without mentioning this important area. Particularly when preparing for a JCAHO survey, the reader should seek details in available relevant references.[6,7]

When Only a Doctor Will Do

Successful implementation of routine systems and resolution of many organizational problems require effective efforts of a leader with a combination of organizational authority, respect of most co-workers, and a reputation for objectivity and fairness. And, in health care, there is an extra dimension. Implementation of many routine systems and resolution of many organizational problems require effective efforts of a leader with a combination of organizational authority, respect of most co-workers, a reputation for objectivity and fairness, and *relevant clinical expertise*. This description often fits a member of the nursing management team.

But beyond that, when one is dealing with physicians, there is a fifth dimension. Many organizational problems are only solved through efforts of a leader with a combination of organizational authority, respect of most co-workers, a reputation for objectivity and fairness, and relevant clinical expertise *who is viewed as a colleague*.

I have often tried to get this point across by role-playing to illustrate the view of many physicians. Putting on my sternest face, I recite my line: "If I were practicing neonatology today, as I once did," goes this role-player line, "and if someone hands me some data or shows me a guideline and tells me I should consider changing the combination of antibiotics I give a newborn with suspected sepsis either to save money or use safer drugs or get a better result for my newborn patient, then the person trying to convince me (expletive) well better be another neonatologist!"

Too many physicians are still arrogant bumblers when trying to express their thoughts and ideas. That line comes across as arrogant, egotistical, and self serving. (If it really is, then use the approach you use with Dr. Yesterday or Dr. Trouble, see page 47.) But the chances are good that this physician is attempting to express a personal and professional concern. In that case, the thought is better expressed like this: "You know, I embrace (or given time and good information can come to accept) changes that must be made for the sake of better results, or the same result achieved in a more efficient manner. But I am responsible for three things as I care for this newborn, and I have to consider them as I consider responding to your request to change my practice habits. The first is that I owe this baby and his parents a reasonably good outcome. The second obligation is something I owe to myself. I deserve to be allowed some professional satisfaction, and, beyond that, I don't need the hassles of a malpractice suit. My third obligation? It is to you (the hospital). You need a good image for successful marketing, and you don't need the hassle of a malpractice suit either. So I need to know you've considered the impact on quality as well as the impact on cost when you make this suggestion. Besides, take a look at my performance record over time. My 'quality data' are good, and my cost data are within established parameters. What is your objection to what I am doing now?" And that takes you into the realm of clinical discussion, which can only be handled by a person with a combination of qualities that include relevant clinical expertise in the area of infectious diseases in high-risk newborns.

The point I have just tried to make is made much better by successful experts in the field of evaluating physician performance, who emphasize that data and valid conclusions are only truly useful if the leadership team includes a network of clinician leaders.[4,8]

The collegial orientation of physicians is likely to be viewed as arrogant cronyism or political strategy by a health care executive who has never been a patient or the family member of a patient. But executives with patient experience have had a chance to observe the professional origins of this collegialism, which is collaborative use of a unique body of knowledge and skills in the context of caring for an individual patient.

By the way, in traditional medical staff models the description of a person with organizational authority, respect, good communication skills, relevant clinical expertise, and status as a colleague of physicians best fits the chair or director of a clinical service and his or her designees. This, in part, explains current insistence by JCAHO that medical staff department chairs or directors be carefully selected, oriented, and evaluated by the medical executive group.

Physicians Are Important at All Organizational Levels

The table on page 14 is a generic summary of roles and responsibilities in any organization. Given a chance, most physicians will choose the role or roles in which they are most comfortable.

It is natural for executives to think of rewarding those who choose to add organizational leadership responsibilities to their clinical responsibilities. If a system is to be successful, physicians (and nurses and other health care professionals) who choose only the frontline worker role must be respected and rewarded as well.[9]

The Executive Edge

Every executive is comfortable relating to people in an organizational context. So relating to physicians who choose roles as physician executives, to board members, or to owners is easy for business-trained members of the management team.

However, relating effectively to clinician leaders and to physicians who choose only the frontline worker role is a unique challenge. Health care executives who meet and master this challenge have an edge in terms of job security and organizational advancement over those who do not.

Discussion Points

1. Is it true that the management style of an effective executive can include sharing leadership? Or is this a sign of weakness that co-workers and subordinates will exploit?

2. Does the governing body of your organization include success in dealing with physicians as a parameter in annual evaluation of the CEO's performance? If not, should the board include this factor in evaluating CEO performance?

   If yes, does this aspect of the evaluation utilize appropriate measurement criteria? Are the measurement criteria fair to the CEO?

3. In your organization, what are some examples of specific issues that require shared leadership? Is credentialing an example? Is shared leadership important in dealing with medical staff issues that arise in the course of mergers and acquisitions?

4. Does the evolution of the position of vice president for medical affairs (VPMA) negate the need to identify and develop clinician leaders?

References

1. Thompson, R. *Health Care Reform as Social Change.* Tampa, Fla.: American College of Physician Executives, 1993.

2. The Atlanta Consulting Group. *America's Health Care: The Big Squeeze.* La Jolla, Calif.: Governance Institute, 1996, p. 2.

3. Merry, M. *The Shifting Quality Focus: Implications for Accreditation and Regulation.* La Jolla, Calif.: Medical Staff Leadership Forum, 1995, p. 8.

4. Mohlenbrock, W. "The Physician Imperative: Define, Measure, and Improve Health Care Quality." *Physician Executive* 24(3):47-54, May-June, 1998.

5. Walton, M. *The Deming Management Method.* New York, N.Y.: Dodd, Mead and Company, 1986, p. 23.

6. *Hospital Accreditation Standards* ("Pocket size" edition). Oakbrook Terrace, Ill.: Joint Commission on Accreditation of Healthcare Organizations, 1998.

7. Thompson, R. *The Compliance Guide to the Medical Staff Standards: Winning Strategies For Your JCAHO Survey*, 2nd Edition. Marblehead, Mass.: Opus Communications, 1998.

8. Garibaldi, R. "Computers and the Quality of Care: A Clinician's Perspective." *New England Journal of Medicine* 338(4):259-60, Jan. 22, 1998.

9. Thompson, R. *So You've Been Integrated, Now What? Opportunities for Physicians Practicing in Managed Care Settings.* Tampa, Fla.: American College of Physician Executives, 1996, p. 23.

ORGANIZATIONAL FUNCTIONS—GENERIC

Worker Function

Technical skills

Best knowledge of product design, production problems, and public reaction.

Frontline interaction with people served by the organization.

Motivated by adequate salary and benefits, but also by pride in one's contribution; satisfaction in a job well-done.

Director/Manager Function

Responsible for dependable performance of one component of the organization/business

- Systems
- Workers
- Documentation
- Evaluation

Executive Function

- Execute
- Assist, guide, support
- Supervise
- External relationships
- On-site governing body authority
- Coordinate

Governance Function

- Ownership
- Fiduciary accountability
- Policies, corporate culture
- Dispute resolution
- Political action
- Community visibility

Chapter 3

Why Shared Leadership Is Difficult—Part 1:
I Didn't Even Know He Sold His House

The new CEO recently came to health care from another industry. Missing a key surgeon at a meeting, the CEO asked the Medical Staff Coordinator if the surgeon would be coming.

"He'll be here," said the coordinator, "but he just called and said he'll be late. He's closing."

"Is that right?" beamed the new CEO. "I didn't even know he sold his house." True story.

Pity the new guy. In his world, "closing" refers to financial transactions. To a surgeon, "closing" means finishing up an operation.

And when the surgeon makes it to the meeting, he may have a similar problem understanding the jargon used by the new chief executive. In one medical staff bylaws revision project, a surgeon objected to a provision that "physicians cooperate with management to the extent necessary to ensure smooth hospital operations." The surgeon thought this language implied some sort of direct control by "administration" over what the surgeon did in the operating room!

Everyone knows how difficult it is for any two people to communicate accurately. In fact, in any interpersonal interaction, mis-communication is the norm.

"I know you believe you understand what you think I said, but I am not sure you realize that what you heard is not what I meant."—**Anonymous**

Many "situation comedy" episodes are based on misdirected or misunderstood personal communications. But, unfortunately, "misunderstandings" are not always funny. Failure of two people to take time to "get on the same wavelength" can result in serious, far-reaching, and long-standing consequences.

The mis-communication problem is accentuated in any situation in which people with disparate training and experience are thrown together and must depend on each other to accomplish a set of tasks.[1] Conscious efforts must continually be exerted to be sure communication is accurate, in terms of both what is being "sent" and what is being "received."

The first step in sharing leadership is: Get acquainted with each other's viewpoints. The table on page 17 lists examples of differences in perspective that must be dealt with openly and honestly.

The first reward of investing the time it takes to communicate accurately is understanding that basic pressures and basic goals are truly shared. Shared goals and pressures include but are not limited to economic success, good public image, the well-deserved self-satisfaction that accompanies accomplishment, providing dependable health care services to beneficiaries and members, and complying with frustrating and complex regulations.

The Added Value of Different Perspectives

The disparate backgrounds of health care executives ("administrators") and physicians was once thought to be a source of inevitable, irreconcilable conflict. But today, while disagreements are a part of any ongoing relationship, members of the leadership team are sharing perspectives, thus creating a powerful coalition. This coalition, which becomes even more powerful as it reaches out to include public leaders and leaders from other industries as well, is well positioned to deal with today's managed care health policy, which encourages profit-taking with one hand while ratcheting down revenues with the other.

Granted, there are too many managed care settings in which the scenario is quite different. In those organizations, executive factions, physician factions, and board factions have allowed the profit-taking health care model to drive deep wedges. In such a setting, there is little hope of experiencing the advantages of shared leadership in the immediate future. These "systems" are bitter battlegrounds in which it is assumed that no one can be a winner until someone else in the same organization is a loser.

Is Your Goal Short-Term or Long-Range?

If your personal goals are short-term, and you have read this far through the book, you are probably guffawing uncontrollably. That's because you know that the "me-only" approach to executive leadership can be successful for a few months or years. And it can be quite lucrative for a small number of individuals. That is, short-term-goal executives can retire young, taking with them significant amounts of money and leaving others to solve the problem of adequately funding health care services.

Characteristics of Executives and Physicians

Executive	Practicing Physician
Trained in and concerned with financial matters (budget, acquisitions, marketing, etc.) group process, personnel management, legalities, external regulations.	Trained in and concerned with disorders in anatomy and/or physiology of the human body—diagnosis and treatment of illness and injury, in a chosen limited clinical field.
Understands that executive privilege is limited by higher authority—governing body policies and organizational goals.	Often appears to believe that there is no higher authority, even , in some instances, The Law.
Data-oriented. Is justifiably concerned with what happens to groups of patients—impact of decisions and actions on the goals of the organization for which the executive has been made responsible by the governing body.	Case-oriented. Is justifiably concerned with what happens to an individual—impact of decisions and actions on the welfare of patients for whom the practitioner is responsible. May not appreciate the value of accumulating and using data, over time.
Responsible for implementing change.	May have Doxology Mentality. "As it was in the beginning, is now and ever shall be."
Must manage to stay within budget, or control costs to maximize profit, depending on the specific health care setting.	May have little experience with planning and limiting expenditures, because of (up to now) large amounts of expendable income.
Delegates responsibilities; goes and does it and reports back.	Fears being "disenfranchised"—don't do anything without asking me first.
Expects to be evaluated.	May view suggestions about how to practice medicine, or even about other matters, as "interference" with a physician's "prerogative."
Allegiance is primarily to the organization employing him or her at the moment, secondarily to others in the same field through colleges, congresses, and associations.	Allegiance is primarily to colleagues through professional relationships and organizations.

The "instant gratification" approach to executive leadership will always have its proponents. But I believe that individuals with this self-serving style will increasingly be passed over by boards of directors, who will favor more mature executives because of boards' interest in staying power, as community leaders (however broad that "community" might be) and/or industrial leaders and as effective fiduciaries for the owners of organizations that the boards govern.[2]

Discussion Points

1. In your business meetings, do members of the leadership group occasionally, on a regular basis, set aside the business agenda for 10 or 15 minutes and remind each other of shared goals?

    If so, do physician members of the leadership team participate effectively in this exercise? Why or why not?

2. In your organization, does the fact that members of the leadership team come from different backgrounds contribute to your strengths? To your weaknesses? Or are the differences insignificant?

3. In your organization, what are some examples of words and phrases that must be carefully defined so that counterproductive misunderstandings can be avoided?

    As a discussion starter, see the Glossary in this book, especially the several uses of the term "managed care."

References

1. Neuhauser, P. Tribal *Warfare in Organizations*. New York, N.Y.: Harper Collins, 1988.

2. Thompson, R. "Sustainability as the Linchpin of Public Policy and Industry Initiatives." *Physician Executive* 24(4):52-5, July-Aug. 1998.

Chapter 4

Why Sharing Leadership Is Difficult—Part 2:
Fifty-Fifty, Like Rabbit Fajitas

On the journey to genuinely shared leadership, we are slowed down by heavy baggage, consisting of unpleasant memories of events long past, long-standing personality conflicts, and hurt feelings that were never healed.

A long history of conflict, distrust, poor communication, and not just a little misunderstanding casts a lingering shadow over attempts by executives, physician leaders, and board members to move forward to the positive era of truly shared leadership.[1-9] It would be a mistake to dwell on history. But a brief mention of past events may prove helpful to the reader for two reasons:

- Men and women who learn some history have a better chance of avoiding unnecessary and sometimes self-defeating mistakes made by their predecessors.

- It is wishful thinking to describe the conflict relationship as all in the past. This is living history with which today's health care executives, so oriented to the future, still must deal.

Bet I Can Hold a Grudge Longer Than You Can

I received a phone call from a CEO who was shopping for a retreat facilitator to help resolve a conflict. I asked if she could give me a brief idea of the nature of the issue. "Well, I've just got a few minutes," she said, "but I'll outline the situation for you." Then there was a long pause as the CEO decided where to start. Finally she began: "Actually this story starts twenty-one years ago, when the administrator that was here then and some doctors who have since retired disagreed on where the new hospital should be built."

The Rabbit Fajitas Joint Venture

At a retreat that I was facilitating, a medical staff president tried to help his bewildered CEO understand why several members of the medical staff chose to oppose a proposed hospital/physician joint adventure.

"A man opened a Mexican restaurant," said the medical staff president, "and started serving rabbit fajitas. An inspector from the County Health Department came around and asked, 'Where are you getting all those rabbits?'"

"Well, to tell the truth," confessed the restaurant owner, "there's a little bit of horsemeat in there. But don't worry, we keep it fifty-fifty. One horse to one rabbit."

Then the medical staff president turned to the CEO and said, "John, that's what some of my colleagues think you mean by working fifty-fifty with your doctors."

The Phone Poll with Still-Relevant Results

The results of a phone poll taken 19 years ago[10] are still relevant in many health care settings. Fifty physicians were asked to say what they thought of "administrators," and 50 "administrators" were asked to describe physicians. As you read the following results, remember that perception is reality, in the sense that it is perception, not reality, that motivates and determines human behavior.

Physicians characterized "hospital administrators" as aloof, insecure bureaucrats concerned with cost accounting but not with patient care, confused about their authority over doctors, and always at bat for the board but never for the physicians. (I heard this view expressed in a retreat within the past six months.)

"Hospital administrators" characterized physicians as egotistical bumblers who resent the superior organizational skills of administrators, are confused about their responsibilities and authority in the hospital, and are above-average people in some ways yet immature and not adept at interpersonal relations.

But also still relevant is the common thread in the comments of both physicians and "hospital administrators" of that day.

But there are two common threads running through some comments of both physicians and "administrators." The two groups agreed that, because administration's responsibility for staying within budget often clashed with physicians' responsibility to do what is necessary to achieve good patient care results, it seemed only natural to expect that disagreements would arise. The other comment made by several doctors and administrators was that it was often possible to work out an amicable compromise to resolve these disagreements, if both organizational communication and individual interpersonal communication are calm, reasonable, and effective.

The Impact of Recent Events

Unfortunately, events of the past five or six years have added a chapter to this history of conflict and distrust.

The result of the Great Health Care Reform Debate of 1993-94 is that "managed care" is cemented in place as the basis of federal and state health care policy. Existing U.S. health

care policy encourages providers to make a profit with one hand, while ratcheting down revenues with the other. Effects of this policy on the executive/physician working relationship vary from location to location.

In some settings, events since 1994 have resulted in development of integrated delivery systems (IDSs) in which a trusting relationship between executives and physicians, and between primary physicians, specialists, and subspecialists, is allowing evolution of true shared leadership and mutual success.

However, seemingly more common is the scenario in which bitter battles over control of "covered lives"; market share; ownership of health care entities, including hospitals and physician practices; and the opportunity to share insurance industry profits have widened the wedge of divisiveness between executives and physicians, and between primary care physicians on one hand and specialists and subspecialists on the other.

We claim to be uncomfortable with conflict. But, in reality, we may be more comfortable with conflict than with the challenge of implementing shared leadership, because conflict is an old friend and shared leadership isn't.

Discussion Points

1. In your organization, are efforts to share leadership obstructed because some individuals are still upset about events that should be past history?

2. If you took a phone poll of a representative sample of medical staff members, what would they say about the management team? What do you think of the physicians on your medical staff (don't over-generalize)?

3. In your organization, what communication mechanisms exist to help physicians understand the problems of the management team? To help the management team understand what's weighing on the minds of physicians?

4. Is it really necessary to work so hard on mutual understanding to build shared leadership? Or is it better to revert to the days when managing the organization and managing patient care were two separate and distinct activities?

References

1. Ponton, T., revised by MacEachern, M. *The Medical Staff in the Hospital*, 2nd Edition. Chicago, Ill.: Physicians Record Company, 1955.

2. Eisele, C., Editor. *The Medical Staff in the Modern Hospital*. New York, N.Y.: McGraw-Hill, 1967.

3. Cunningham, R. *Governing Hospitals: Trustees and the New Accountabilities*. Chicago, Ill.: American Hospital Association, 1976, pp. 88-92.

4. Thompson, R. *Helping Hospital Trustees Understand Physicians*. Chicago, Ill.: American Hospital Association, 1979.

5. Cadmus, R. *Hospitals Are Us*. Chicago, Ill.: Teach 'Em, 1979.

6. Thompson, R. *Physicians and Hospitals: Easing Adversary Relationships*. Chicago, Ill.: Pluribus Press, 1984.

7. Eisele, C., and others. *The Medical Staff and the Modern Hospital*. Englewood, Colo.: Estes Park Institute, 1985.

8. Shortell, S. *Effective Hospital-Physician Relationships*. Chicago, Ill.: Health Administration Press, 1991.

9. Flynn, D. "How Much is That CEO in the Window?" *Healthcare Executive* 6(1):28-9, Jan.-Feb. 1991.

10. "Cooperation or Conflict: Physicians vs. Administrators." *Hospitals* 53(14):72-5, July 16, 1979.

Chapter 5

Why Sharing Leadership Is Difficult—Part 3: Who's in Charge?

Shared leadership only works when both responsibility and authority, and their limits, are first carefully defined.

Even in familiar areas, such as privileging and caring for individual patients, the exercise of defining relative roles is not yet fully completed.

"Who's in charge around here?"

Inexperienced executives and managers will try to answer that question by referring to an organizational chart. But experienced executives and managers know what's between the lines and boxes and arrows on that organizational diagram.

For one thing, people in authority sometimes have less control than a person without much official clout whose influence prevails because of the power to persuade. Also, an individual's authority and responsibility may need to be described in the context of a specific organizational task.

So the global question, "Who's in charge?" is really impossible to answer. The question must be stated as, "Who's in charge of what?" Perhaps that's true in any organization. At the very least, it is a critical guiding principle when working with physician leaders and frontline clinical practitioners.

Here are four examples of relative roles described in the context of a specific organizational task.

Creating an Annual Budget for the Organization

The chief financial officer (CFO), with delegated authority from the CEO and board, takes the point in creating and proposing a budget.

It is the prerogative and obligation of relevant physician leaders, nursing leaders, and department directors to provide accurate assessments of budgetary needs when asked to do so. For example, the vice president of medical affairs (VPMA) should be asked for, and should provide, overall guidance in areas of the budget related to physician services promised by the organization and with respect to the budget for operation of the office of the VPMA. The VPMA should seek input from the coordinator of the medical staff office regarding that office's budgetary needs, including systemwide credentialing, and should provide that input to the CFO.

The CEO and CFO must present the budget to the board, whose job it is to finalize and approve next year's budget.

Note that there is no need for the medical executive committee to take any formal part in creating the organization's budget at either the hospital level or the system level. In addition, while medical executive functions would include responsibility (borrowing authority delegated by the board) for evaluating the dependability of clinical performance of contracted physicians and/or physician groups, it is not usual or necessary for the medical executive committee to be involved in details of salary and other contract arrangements with contracted physicians.

Preparing and Safeguarding Medical Records

The various portions of the patients' medical record are completed by clinical professionals whose contributions to the patient's care are reflected in that area of the record. For example, results of laboratory tests are recorded by laboratory personnel, delivered to the clinical care unit, and posted by unit clerical personnel. It is the prerogative and obligation of the attending physician to complete the summary information "face sheet" of a hospitalized patient's medical record. And the portion of the hospitalized patient's record reflecting nursing care functions is completed by nurses.

It is the responsibility of the director and the staff of the information services department (including the medical records division) to obtain entries from responsible individuals to "complete" the medical record. In the hospital component of the IDS, it is traditional for patients' medical records (a critical document for the hospital, the system, and the patients' physicians as well as for the patient) to lie incomplete for weeks. That's because, at this writing, it is still the attending physician's prerogative to complete the "face sheet" of the medical record, at his or her convenience.

Long delay in completing patients' medical records is unacceptable. It's true that some portions of the record, such as the "face sheet" summary of "final diagnoses" and the "discharge summary," cannot be completed until the results of hospitalization are known. But in hospitals where shared leadership works, the executive staff mandates joint efforts of physician leaders and the medical records division of the information services department to improve systems for completing patient records so that long delays do not occur. Besides, for some parts of the patient's record, traditional delays are unnecessary. Physicians' signatures and, of course, current "progress notes" should really be completed during the care of the hospitalized patient.

With respect to getting needed entries from physicians, such as final diagnoses and signatures, medical records personnel borrow authority delegated by physician leaders and the board through the medical staff bylaws.

Access to patients' medical records is governed by a release of information policy, prepared by the director of information services, reviewed by relevant legal counsel, and approved by the board.

Note that the CEO, in spite of his or her high position on the "organizational chart," is not ordinarily authorized to write entries in the medical records.

Credentialing and Privileging Independent Practitioners

Even with a system as familiar as credentialing and privileging, the exercise of breaking the system down into individual sequential tasks (taking care not to skip any) can be surprisingly valuable. Responsible individuals can gain improved understanding of the purpose of each step and of the need for interaction between participants in the process.

In the Hospital

Confirming entry-level qualifications of independent clinical practitioners (ICPs) is probably the most widely recognized example of shared leadership. The confirmation system is activated when an individual requests an application form. The form, which has been approved by the medical executive committee and by the board or relevant board committee, is provided to the requestor, or not, by medical staff office personnel, using rules and guidelines established and approved by the board.

When an applicant returns initially requested information, it is sorted, compiled in a file, and verified by medical staff office and/or credentialing office personnel.

This preliminary file must then be *read* by the board chair or a duly constituted representative, such as the CEO or the VPMA. The completed file is also *read* by the medical staff president or his designee, such as the VPMA, the chair of the credentials committee if there is one, or a physician knowledgeable about the credentialing and privileging process.

These individuals, working in concert, either declare the application "complete" (ready for the next step in processing) or give the medical staff/credentialing office a list of additional information items needed to adequately evaluate the applicant.

In the latter event, it is the responsibility of the medical staff coordinator to request this information from the applicant. It is the responsibility of the applicant to provide it. (Credentialing rules should state that, if the applicant chooses not to accomplish this step, no further processing of the application is required.)

If, at any point in this process, the individuals responsible for reading the application have questions they would like to ask the applicant, they should call (or delegate the medical staff coordinator to call), ask their questions, objectively record the answers using as near to the applicant's own language as possible, and attach this documentation to the application.

When the individuals responsible for *reading* the application are satisfied that all information necessary for the *credentialing* step (the *privileging* step requires consideration of detailed information about clinical qualifications and experience) has been provided and validated, they declare the application "complete" and affix their signatures to a memo so stating, a copy of which is sent to the applicant by the medical staff coordinator.

Upon receiving notification that the application is complete, the applicant is entitled to expect that notification of action on the application will not be far behind.

Now the relevant clinical department chair (the chair of the clinical department to which the applicant will be assigned if granted membership and/or clinical privileges) officially enters the picture. Clinical department chairs are especially oriented to review that portion of an application related to privileging. The question to which the chair is expected to respond is, "Does it appear to you that the training, experience, and current dependability of performance of this applicant match the clinical privileges being requested?"

The completed application, plus the department chair's report (whether positive or negative), then go forward to the medical executive committee level (in older organizational models, through a credentials subcommittee to the medical executive committee). The medical executive or medical executive group and CEO frame a recommendation for action on the application. The CEO or VPMA presents a summary of information about the application, plus the recommendation, to the board of directors/trustees or to the relevant board committee. It is the board's prerogative and responsibility to either appoint or disappoint the applicant.

Note that there is no routine role for attorneys in the processing of applications. Rather, the role of the organization's attorney is to evaluate the credentialing and privileging system when it is established by the medical executive committee and board to be sure

that the system satisfies any relevant federal and state laws and/or regulations, and to advise the organization's leadership of any relevant legal precedents of which they should be aware.

In addition, the attorney should be "on call" for early consultation in the event an individual's application appears to be something other than routine.

At the Integrated System/Network Level

Accurate understanding and effective implementation of the sequential tasks in hospital credentialing are very helpful in avoiding duplicate effort and needless conflicts in systemwide credentialing (see figure on page 32[1]).

The Ultimate Example of Needing Careful Clarification of Responsibilities: Clinical Care of Each Individual Patient

Some executives may be surprised to learn that clinical professionals still need prodding from senior management as an incentive to communicate with one another about where the responsibility of one ends and the responsibility of another begins. Clearer explanations are not enough. Senior managers must make sure that caregivers hear each other's explanations clearly and govern their activities accordingly.

Rewards of this exercise can include reduced costs of care, enhanced public image, and avoidance of unnecessary legal problems—not to mention more dependable care for each patient, client, and resident!

A Brief Example

Here is a brief example of clarification of relative roles and responsibilities in the context of caring for an individual patient.

The Patient

An individual sets our clinical systems in motion when he or she decides that a medical problem has reached the point of requiring professional attention. For any illness, this decision may be made at the onset of early mild symptoms or not until the appearance of complications. The decision by a person to become a "patient" is a primary determinant of "severity of illness" at the time of entry into the health care system.

Physician Roles and Responsibilities

The first physician who evaluates and "attends" this patient becomes the practitioner primarily responsible for whatever happens next. The physician might determine that he or she can diagnose and treat the patient without consultation or might seek clinical consultation on an outpatient basis. Or the "primary attending" might order hospitalization ("admit" the patient) and continue to attend the patient in the hospital or might admit the patient and seek clinical consultation from other physicians who work in the hospital.

If clinical consultation is ordered, it is the obligation of the primary attending physician to decide whether the clinical consultant is to see the patient only once for evaluation and to make recommendations about the care plan, is to "follow the patient with" the primary attending physician, or is to assume primary responsibility for care of the patient.

Failure of the primary attending physician and consulting physicians to accept responsibility for communicating accurately and effectively with one another and with members of the nursing staff can be a major issue in medical malpractice cases, to the detriment of the hospital as well as of the individual practitioners involved.

Now, if our "patient" has a "surgical problem," a surgical specialist may be added to this picture. If an operation is indeed necessary, a team of "operating surgeons" may be the same as or may be different from the attending and consulting physicians already attending the patient, and the services of an anesthesiologist will be needed. It is the prerogative and responsibility of the operating surgeon and the anesthesiologist to care for the patient in the immediate preoperative period, the "recovery period," and the immediate postoperative period and to communicate with each other and with nurses caring for the patient to clarify which physician is (or physicians are) assuming order-writing authority in each phase of the patient's care.

Physician Roles Continued: Understanding Why Practice Guidelines Are Not Enough

"Clinical decision making" is the process of tailoring "practice guidelines" to fit a patient's individual needs. At this writing, this is still the prerogative of physicians. This individualization of diagnostic and treatment plans is truly necessary. Think about it this way:

Have you ever noticed a stranger who bears a close resemblance to a friend or relative? If so, think about your reaction, which usually is something like, "Wow, isn't that amazing!

He looks almost exactly like Bill." In other words, while facial features have certain standardized characteristics (there's an ear on each side of the head, a nose in the middle of the face, and a mouth somewhere down around a chin that may be either prominent or recessed), the *specifics* of facial characteristics are so unique and individualized that it is a rarity to encounter look-alikes. We are well aware of this and accept this fact without even thinking about it.

So we must now realize that a person's physiologic characteristics; temperamental make-up; ability to stand pain; and previous experiences with health, accidents, and disease are as unique as his or her facial characteristics. This fact will make clinical decision making a necessary skill, even in a future era when clinical practice guidelines are sophisticated and universally accepted.

Nursing Roles and Responsibilities
Meanwhile, a number of nurses in both the outpatient and inpatient settings are accepting responsibility for meeting needs of the patient related to services ordinarily accepted as "nursing services." When I was a hospitalized patient, I told my nurses with a twinkle in my eye that they seemed preoccupied with the Four B's. Those were bed, bath, blood pressure, and bowels. Just for spite, they really should have left me totally unattended in all those areas!

A person who becomes a patient suddenly finds him- or herself dependent, to a greater or lesser degree, on nursing care handled by nurses of various skill levels. But responsibility and authority of nursing in the context of caring for a patient is much, much more than care of bodily functions!

Nurses assess the social circumstances from which a patient comes and to which he or she will return; observe and interpret monitors of heart rate, blood pressure, respirations, and other "vital signs"; see to the comfort of family members (both in the sense of bodily comfort and in the sense of inspiring confidence that the patient is receiving good care); coordinate with the staff of departments such as radiology and laboratory to secure needed diagnostic tests and their results in a timely manner; dress surgical wounds;

provide patient education (and often physician education!); motivate the patient to comply with physicians' instructions, such as self-performed rehabilitating exercises and self-administration of medications; and participate in discharge planning.

Roles and Responsibilities of Clinical Technicians
The doctors and nurses caring for a hospitalized patient (not to mention the patient!) are dependent on clinical technicians of several disciplines who provide a variety of skilled services. These services range from performing radiological, imaging, and laboratory studies to pharmaceutical services, rehabilitation services, etc.

This Clinical Team Must Communicate!

It is the responsibility of members of this "patient care team" to communicate effectively with one another regarding responsibilities and authority that each assumes and that each expects others to assume. And it is primarily the physician's responsibility to avoid leaving too much up to other members of this patient care team.

For example, some physicians tend to rely too much on nurses and technicians to secure "informed consent" from patients. The goal of informed consent is to give the patient (or a surrogate in some situations) the information needed to make a prudent choice from several available options, including no treatment at all.[2] It is now widely accepted that "adequate informed consent requires effort on the part of the physician to require comprehension."[3]

Note that the CEO is not authorized (by state licensure and or by "privileging") to participate in or make suggestions about the care of individual patients. Yet it is the cost and results of such care, reflected in accumulated outcome statistics and financial reports, that determine whether the board's evaluation of the CEO is favorable or unfavorable.

Note also that executives who attempt to participate in the care of individual patients, such as by implementing rules restricting what patients may be told and/or what services patients may be offered, are simultaneously endangering the health of the patient, the reputation and professional satisfaction of doctors and nurses responsible for this patient, and the integrity of the organization, and thus also the organization's public image.

Discussion Points

1. In your organization, is it possible to name one individual or group in response to the question, "Who's in charge?" If so, who is this person, or which group can be so named?

2. Does your credentialing and privileging guidelines and policies manual include a straightforward description of everyone's role in the process, similar to the example given in this chapter? If not, should you create such a description? If you should, who should be in charge of accomplishing this task? (Use the example in this chapter to guide your thinking, but do not photocopy and adopt it. Rather discuss, modify, and adapt it as needed. Remember that your description must match existing provisions of medical staff bylaws and related documents.)

3. When a merger or acquisition is considered, or if hospital executive staff members and the board consider selling the hospital or becoming part of another system, at what point should physician leaders and frontline practitioners learn about these plans? At what point should physician leaders be dropped from the final decision-making process?

4. In your organization's "performance improvement" efforts to maintain and improve clinical care systems, are there any systems that might benefit from the type of "task analysis" demonstrated in the four examples in this chapter?

5. Pretend you are the patient. List three clinical systems that must work effectively if you are to receive dependable care. (Example: timely administration of ordered medications.) Break each of the clinical care systems you have listed into a list of sequential tasks. Be sure you have not omitted any necessary tasks.

Now answer the question, "Who's in charge?" for each of these tasks.

Consider preserving the results of this exercise as beginning pages of a guidelines manual entitled:

WHO'S IN CHARGE OF WHAT?
Clarification of Relevant Responsibility and Authority
for Several Key Clinical Systems

References

1. Thompson, R. *So You've Been Integrated, Now What? Opportunities for Physicians Practicing in Managed Care Organizations.* Tampa, Fla.: American College of Physician Executives, 1996, p. 57.

2. Junkerman, C., and Schiedermayer, D. *Practical Ethics for Students, Interns, and Residents:* A Short Reference Manual. Frederick, Md.: University Publishing Group, Inc., 1998, p. 13.

3. President's Commission for the Study of Ethical Problems in Medicine and Biomedical and Behavioral Research. *Making Health Care Decisions: The Ethical and Legal Implications of Informed Consent on the Patient-Physician Relationship.* Washington, D.C.: U.S. Government Printing Office, 1982.

Schematic Presentation of Credentialing Process in an Integrated Delivery System

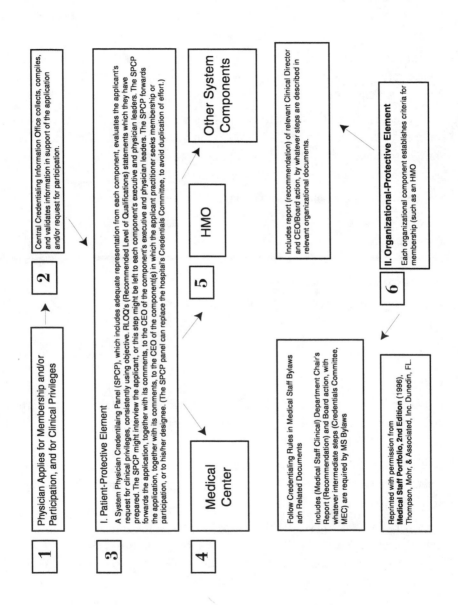

1 Physician Applies for Membership and/or Participation, and for Clinical Privileges

2 Central Credentialing Information Office collects, compiles, and validates information in support of the application and/or request for participation.

3 I. Patient-Protective Element

A System Physician Credentialing Panel (SPCP), which includes adequate representation from each component, evaluates the applicant's request for clinical privileges, consistently using objective. RLOQs (Recommended Level of Qualifications) statements which they have prepared. The SPCP might interview the applicant, or this step might be left to each component's executive and physician leaders. The SPCP forwards the application, together with its comments, to the CEO of the component's executive and physician leaders. The SPCP forwards the application, together with its comments, to the CEO of the component(s) in which the applicant practitioner seeks membership or participation, or to his/her designee. (The SPCP panel can replace the hospital's Credentials Committee, to avoid duplication of effort.)

4 Medical Center

Follow Credentialing Rules in Medical Staff Bylaws adn Related Documents

Includes (Medical Staff Clinical) Department Chair's Report (Recommendation) and Board action, with whatever intermediate steps (Credentials Committee, MEC) are required by MS Bylaws

5 HMO

6 II. Organizational-Protective Element

Each organizational component establishes criteria for membership (such as an HMO

Other System Components

Includes report (recommendation) of relevant Clinical Director and CEO/Board action, by whatever steps are described in relevant organizational documents.

Reprinted with permission from **Medical Staff Portfolio, 2nd Edition** (1996), Thompson, Mohr, & Associated, Inc. Dunedin, FL.

Chapter 6
Why Sharing Leadership Is Difficult—Part 4: Managed Care's Ethical Immaturity

Shared leadership cannot happen when the business ethic of executives differs markedly from the professional ethic of frontline professionals who provide the services promised by the organization.

I am not a formally trained ethicist and do not represent myself as such. But I believe that we should not leave ethical considerations totally in the hands of academic ethicists, just as ethicists believe that the health care business should not be left totally in the hands of executives, politicians, bankers, and doctors.

Those of us in the "health care operations" world must be able to think clearly about ethical issues for two reasons:

- The ethical maturity of an academic ethicist is of no value to people in need of health care services if those making health care management decisions (and health care public policy decisions) are ethically immature.

- Failure to develop a shared ethic is a major stumbling block to the evolution of shared leadership between executives and physicians.

What Does It Mean to Be Ethical?

He's such a strange man. He doesn't seem to know what's right, only what's legal.—Agatha Christie.

An ethic is a personal code that motivates a person's plans, decisions, and actions (behavior). This ethic arises from a set of values. Values are personal beliefs about what is and is not important. Values are developed over time, beginning in childhood, as a result of a variety of influences. Part of each person's value system is whether or not the rights of others are respected. A right is something that an individual can reasonably expect to receive, based on a justifiable claim. That claim may be based on tradition and experience (a customary right), on the law and government (legal rights and civil rights), or simply on the existence of the individual as a human being (human rights).

Some ethicists use the words "ethics" and "morality" interchangeably, but clarify that moral is not synonymous with good versus evil or with puritanical prohibitions.[1]

One school of ethical thought suggests that a person's behavior should be guided by a set of rules that should be universally and absolutely applied to all situations encountered by the individual. Another school of thought suggests that what is ethical should be determined by using logic and reason to apply one's value system to given issues and circumstances.

An ethical dilemma exists when the rights of two or more individuals or groups are in conflict, so that there is no absolutely "right" approach either in the sense of "logically correct" or "morally good." That's because more than one set of values apply to the situation.

Ethics, philosophy, and religion are closely related. Ethics is one of the five branches of philosophy. One feature of a religion is that its followers display an ethic governed by the doctrines and the rules of the religion.

One purpose of laws and regulations is to protect people from invasion of their rights by people whose ethic is one of an extreme degree of economic self-interest.

A corporate ethic (popularly referred to as an organization's corporate culture) reflects the personal ethic of those in charge of plans, decisions, and actions of the corporation.

What Is Ethical Immaturity?

There are several varieties of ethical immaturity. One is failing to define and/or accept a set of values at all. Another type of ethical immaturity is failing to use logic and reason to apply defined value systems to determine what is and is not ethical behavior. This is often the result of not knowing how to frame or state an ethical question or a set of ethical questions. Or one may not know how to use "mentally methodological approaches"[2] (how to think!) to resolve ethical dilemmas.

For example, managed care is criticized because, as succinctly summarized by Junkerman and Schiedermayer, "more than $50 billion was generated as profits in health care in 1997, while policymakers solemnly agree that we can't afford universal health care."[3] If this circumstance had been created as a result of applying reason and logic to the ethical dilemma of profit versus service, it would not be ethical immaturity because one possible choice of an ethic is self-gratification. But, in actuality, this outcome is simply the composite of a series of actions by policy makers, legislators, and managed care organizations whose "reasoning" has so far been focused only on health care financing and profit. That is ethical immaturity.

Here are some additional examples intended to help the reader better understand the concept of ethical maturity vs. ethical immaturity.

Example 1: The Word of God, As Spoken Directly to Me

Some vehicles display a bumper sticker that says, "God Spoke It. I Believe It. That Settles It."

As mentioned above, obeying a religious code can be a sign of ethical maturity. However, some of the "religious right" owners of vehicles bearing this bumper sticker appear to exhibit ethically immature behavior. For example a TV repairman, after repairing a relative's TV set, advised her that he had "fixed it" so she could now receive a "religious channel" that this TV repairman recommended. Thus it seems that his religious code prohibiting stealing was laid aside in the case of pirating a TV signal to further his religious cause.

Or a single individual may support family values and oppose "sin," including murder, but at the same time see bombing an abortion clinic as a good way to defend and protect (this individual's interpretation of) family values and the sanctity of human life.

Such behavior is quite different from a more moderate interpretation of choosing to obey a religious code.

Example 2: Learning to Apply Personal Value Systems Using Logic and Reason

Is it any wonder that those of us working in health care are ethically immature, in the sense of not having experience in applying logic and reason, when today the most common "buzzword" guiding our behavior (and limiting our development!) is "compliance?"

The following example demonstrates learning to use logic and reason as an approach to developing ethical maturity.[4]

As a class exercise, a group of agricultural students were asked to assume an imaginary situation. They were to pretend that a new drug is available that has the same effect as steroids but that cannot be detected by any blood or urine test. (In the real world, there is a rule that prohibits giving steroids to a show animal in order to increase the animal's chance of winning the blue ribbon.) The students were then asked to discuss whether or not they would give the imaginary new wonder drug to their show animals.

Some students chose not to use the drug because of an innate sense of "fairness," because they were concerned about possible problems that the animal might experience from taking the drug, or because they felt that such artificial enhancement of their animal's desirable characteristics would interfere with the true spirit of the competition.

Other students chose to use the drug because they figured others would be using it, making it fair for them to use it, because they reasoned that medical complications in an animal intended for slaughter should not be considered of great significance, and because they wished to give the proceeds from selling a blue ribbon animal to their parents in return for the expense of helping them through college.

Note three (at least) things about this example.

First, although the decision of one group of students or the other will surely seem "wrong" or "bad" to some, both decisions can be considered ethical behavior if each student really knows his or her value system and applied it honestly to this ethical dilemma.

Second, note the value (in terms of learning to apply logic and reason) of setting up a situation in which the fear of being "caught" is eliminated.

Third, notice that accurately stating an ethical question (whether for an educational exercise or in the operation of a business) is itself a skill that must be learned and practiced. For example, Professor Thompson purposely posed this practice dilemma in such a way that cost was not a primary issue. So the students did not contaminate their discussions and decisions with questions of financial feasibility. The students who chose not to use such a drug need never deal with the question of cost. The other group, having decided it is ethical to use the drug, would (in the real world) now have to proceed to the question of financial feasibility.

In relation to health care policy, note that the Great Health Care Reform Debate of 1993-94 was all about the mechanism of financing health care, without any preceding discussions leading to agreement, stated as a matter of uniform policy, about how much of what kinds of health care should be offered to whom.

An ethically mature approach to establishing health care policy would involve simultaneous consideration of at least four factors:

- Definition of the amount of health care (if any) to which all U.S. citizens are entitled.
- Delivery system options related to users' needs.
- Measurement of dependable performance from the standpoint of both users and payers.
- Feasible options for financing the system that has been defined by consideration of the other three issues.[5]

Example 3: Euthanasia

Euthanasia (from the Greek *eu-* easy + *thanatos* death) is a good example of an ethical dilemma faced by health care providers and policy makers and by lawmakers. Several conclusions about this issue are logical, and none of them are unethical. The reader interested in studying the euthanasia issue in depth is referred to the internet site, www.euthanasia.com,[6] which at this writing lists 164 articles and resources.

One approach to euthanasia is to follow the code of a chosen religion, if that religion's doctrine includes a rule concerning euthanasia.

Another approach is to follow the code of civil law. Some countries, notably Australia and the Netherlands, have experimented with legal euthanasia and so has the state of Oregon. In addition, some studies suggest that, while Dr. Kevorkian stands alone in openly defying federal and state prohibitions against euthanasia, well-meaning physicians and nurses may occasionally respond to pleas from patients to hurry along a perceived inevitable death.[7,8] The occasional horror story about an intensive care unit nurse or long-term-care facility employee who performs mercy killing using his or her own judgment about who should die right now and who shouldn't, and who acts without a patient's prior knowledge, is, of course, an entirely different issue.

Still another approach to euthanasia might be classified as utilitarian by an ethicist. Proponents of this approach argue for a form of rationing medical care services based on age, so that limited health care dollars can be distributed more fairly to provide clinical services to people of all ages and with all types of medical and surgical problems.[9] One caution voiced by some is that "the age-based rationing debate has captured our attention because it promises a quick fix for the problem of financing health care...(which is misleading because)...philosophers do us a service by stimulating public debate, but...have little to contribute to detailed resolution of problems (which) inevitably involves political negotiation, compromise, and a level of practical judgment that eludes pure theory."[10]

This sounds like validation of the argument that those with power to make decisions about the availability, the dependability and the cost of health care resources must take time to engage in relevant ethical debates in an attempt to include rational ethical considerations in "practical judgments" related to framing health care policy.[5]

Finally, some people's value systems motivate them (consciously or unconsciously) to focus on the right of an individual to choose a dignified and relatively painless death at a time selected by the individual. Proponents of this approach include famous people known to be ethically mature.[10]

One of the greatest medical teachers of all time, Sir William Osler of Johns Hopkins University, was heavily criticized in his mature years for appearing to champion a planned life with a "fixed period" of duration in his farewell address to his Johns Hopkins colleagues.[11] Osler later claimed that his reference to a "planned life" meant only that the prestigious position that he was leaving Johns Hopkins to assume was one for which his professional studies and accomplishments had prepared him. Furthermore, he said, his reference to a "fixed period" lifetime was merely an attempt at humor, a reference to a farcical novel by Victorian writer Anthony Trollope.[12] Trollope's novel depicts an imaginary country in which everyone is admitted to a "college" on their 67th birthday for a year of intense preparation for euthanasia by chloroform on their 68th birthday. Still, newspapers continued to scream, "Osler Recommends Chloroform at Sixty!" Unfortunately, this furor resulted in cancellations of pledges by donors to Johns Hopkins University.

So apparently the issue of euthanasia was as clouded by raging emotions and knee-jerk reporting as it is today. A discussion of euthanasia in which several alternatives are calmly discussed, and in which disparate views are respected, requires a very high level of ethical maturity.

The participation of health care providers and professionals is needed in the euthanasia debate. But some wonder if they can trust us to participate objectively in the debate as long as U.S. health care policy encourages "doing what it takes" to maximize investor profit.

For example, one basic business principle is "cut the losers." The chronically ill, the acutely but irreversibly ill, and elderly people are definitely money-losers for the health care system.

Why would it not be appropriate to suspect that "managed care's" approach to euthanasia discussions would be based on the self-serving ethic that has developed by default in an ethically immature system?

Relevance to Shared Leadership

Until executives and physicians make a conscious effort to develop and acknowledge a shared ethic that effectively balances profit with service, truly shared leadership will not happen.

The investor-profit ethic and the professional ethic are bound to be at odds in today's era of expensive medical technology combined with a patchwork national health care policy that encourages profit-taking with one hand while ratcheting down payments to providers and professionals with the other.[13-15]

Some in the health care business defend and live by the "whatever it takes to maximize profit" ethic. Others in the health care business have a professional ethic of "deliver dependable clinical services within budget, which budget may or may not include reasonable profit depending on the legal structure of the organization." Some people seem surprised to discover that there are executives and physicians among the champions of both these views of "business!"

Some obstructions to evolution of truly shared leadership are not clearly and simply a matter of "executives" versus "physicians."

Discussion Points

1. In your organization, have executives and physician leaders worked together to create a shared ethic? If so, what is the name of the document in which this ethic is recorded? What efforts have been made to achieve buy-in to this shared ethic on the part of frontline practicing clinicians?

2. Name three recent plans, decisions, or actions of the executive staff that were made or taken because of reference to the shared ethic referred to in #1 above.

3. Name three recent plans, decisions, or actions of the executive staff that were made or taken without reference to the shared ethic referred to in #1.

4. Name three recent plans, decisions, or actions of the executive staff that were made in conscious violation of the shared ethic referred to in #1 above.

5. Given the results of discussing questions 2, 3, and 4, what is your conclusion regarding the degree of agreement or conflict between your shared ethic and your operational decisions?

6. Given the results of discussing questions 1, 2, 3, 4, and 5, what is your estimate of the ethical maturity of the leaders of your organization?

7. Is ethical maturity possible in the investor/profit-taking model for financing integrated delivery of clinical services?

References

1. Singer, P. *Practical Ethics*, Second Edition. New York, N.Y.: Cambridge University Press, 1993.

2. Worthley, J. *The Ethics of the Ordinary in Healthcare: Concepts and Cases.* Chicago, Ill.: Health Administration Press, 1997, p. 199.

3. Junkerman, C., and Schiedermayer, D. *Practical Ethics for Students, Interns, and Residents.* Frederick, Md.: University Publishing Group, Inc., 1998, p. 52.

4. Thompson, P. Class Exercise. When this class exercise was observed, Dr. Thompson was Director of the Institute on Policy and Ethics in Biotechnology at Texas A&M University, College Station, Texas. He is now Joyce and Edward E. Brewer Distinguished Professor of Applied Ethics, Purdue University, West Lafayette, Indiana.

5. Thompson, R. "Sustainability as the Linchpin of Public Policy and Industry Initiatives." *Physician Executive* 24(4):52-5, July/Aug. 1998.

6. www.euthanasia.com. Specific references change periodically as this list of articles and resources is updated.

7. Meier, D., and others. "A National Survey of Physician-Assisted Suicide and Euthanasia in the United States." *New England Journal of Medicine* 338(17):1193-1201, April 23, 1998.

8. Asch, D. "The Role of Critical Care Nurses in Euthanasia and Assisted Suicide." *New England Journal of Medicine* 334(21):1374-9, May 23, 1996.

9. Callahan, D. *Setting Limits: Medical Goals in an Aging Society, With a Response to My Critics*, Second Edition. Washington, D.C.: Georgetown University Press, 1995.

10. Moody, Harry R. *Ethics in an Aging Society*. Baltimore, Md.: Johns Hopkins University Press, 1992, p. 207.

11. Johnson, H. "Osler Recommends Chloroform at Sixty." *The Pharos: Journal of the Alpha Omega Alpha Honor Medical Society* 59(1):24, Winter 1996.

12. Trollope, A. *The Fixed Period* (originally published in 1882). London, England: Penguin Books, 1993.

13. Thompson, R. *Health Care Reform as Social Change.* Tampa, Fla.: American College

of Physician Executives, 1993, pp. ii-iv.

14. Kassirer, J. "Managing Care: Should We Adopt a New Ethic?" *New England Journal of Medicine* 339(6):397-8, Aug. 6, 1998.

15. Shortell, S., and others. "Policy Perspectives: Physicians as double agents. Maintaining trust in an era of multiple accountabillities." *JAMA* 280(12):1102-8, Sept.23-30, 1998.

Chapter 7

Why Sharing Leadership Is Difficult—Part 5: Leading Is Harder Than Managing

Leadership is about achieving goals.—Garry Wills[1]

A 1990s political cartoonist once depicted a group of friendly aliens, with their recently landed spaceship in the background, conversing with an earthling in his backyard. "Well, then," the aliens are asking, "how long do you think it will take for a clear leader to emerge?"

This cartoon reflects the fact that a dependable and trustworthy leader is today a rare and valuable commodity. One reason is that there has been little appreciation in recent years of the difference between leading and managing. (For a list of some differences between leadership and management, see table 1, page 47.)

Low Risk "Leaders"

One reason for a shortage of true leaders in government and on management teams is that true leaders risk controversy and criticism when they urge disciplined and coordinated effort focused on achieving a clearly stated goal. Managers take no such risks. Indeed, a good manager knows many techniques for avoiding decision making and its attendant risks. For example, everybody knows what "CYA" stands for.

The most common technique for avoiding the risks and the responsibilities of decision making is to call in a consultant or an attorney or both to make decisions, and let them take any ensuing consequences. By the way, managers who operate in this way are among the loudest complainers about the fact that too many decisions are being made these days by attorneys and consultants.

Finally, Physician Leaders Emerge

Finding a good organizational leader among a group of physicians was, until just a few years ago, like trying to find a needle in a haystack. In fact, some considered the phrase "physician leader" an oxymoron! At least five factors have delayed development of true physician leadership in health care organizations:

1. *The nature of a physician's work is acceptance of clinical responsibility, which is not something that can be easily delegated.* For several reasons, it isn't wise for a surgeon to schedule an operation and then send somebody else to perform the operation in his or her name. Because of the nature of clinical responsibility (plus in some instances because of innate bullheadedness), two or more physicians attending, consulting, and/or operating on a single patient may not even share leadership and decision making graciously among themselves. So, the organizational skill of delegating specific tasks does not come naturally to many physicians.

2. *Traditionally thinking physicians often do not distinguish political leadership from organizational leadership.* A political leader is a position-taker, whereas an organizational leader is a problem-solver. A political leader is usually responsible for protecting the status of a "constituency," whereas a leadership team in a health care organization must work together to deliver dependable clinical services at reasonable cost and in a timely manner.

3. *Sometimes, executives and managers delayed development of physician leadership by wanting every doctor to become a manager.* Today, management teams better understand the role of physicians on the leadership team. That is, a physician leader who learns enough organizational skills to be a good chair or director of a clinical service is also valued as a frontline practitioner, not encouraged to get an MBA degree.

4. *Physician appreciation of organizational skills is a relatively recent development.* Many physicians today understand the difference between clinical skills, such as diagnosing and operating, and organizational skills, such as communicating effectively and running meetings that start on time, end on time, and accomplish something. But, to this day, when I'm first introduced to a physician group to speak or consult, at least one or two physicians in the group want to know, "Do you still practice?" Between the lines, they really want to know, "Do you understand enough about what we do that we can trust and depend on your information and leadership?"

   Often this is a friendly inquiry. So I answer in good humor, such as "No, I'm like John Madden. He doesn't play or coach football anymore, but he still understands the game and the players so he's welcome in the locker room."

   But sometimes the questioner's demeanor suggests that he or she is thinking something like, "If I don't like what this guy says, tomorrow, after he's left, I can discredit him with my colleagues by pointing out that he doesn't even practice anymore." In that case, I answer seriously: "No, I don't practice pediatrics anymore. And you should be glad. Given the situation you are trying to deal with, you don't need someone with clinical skills. You need someone with organizational skills. That's why your leaders selected me."

5. *Some physicians still tend to be suspicious of leaders who become too effective, even when the medical staff chooses its own leaders.* "Maybe we shouldn't have elected John," a group of physicians may say. "Looks to me like he's gone over to the other side."

That's why, in #4 above, I had to carefully say, "Your leaders selected me." I couldn't say, "That's why you selected me." I made the mistake of doing that once, and I was immediately pounced on by the questioner. "I didn't select you!" he exclaimed triumphantly. "They selected you!"

As one physician put it, "We don't think vertically, Dick. We think horizontally." That means physicians tend to think in terms of "leaders and colleagues," rather than in terms of "leaders and followers." The view of the questioner in the preceding example was that "they" are the leadership team that selected me, and "we," to him, meant "those of us they disenfranchised by not letting us vote on which consultant to select."

With that kind of "followship," it was hard for interested and committed physician leaders to develop their leadership skills.

The key to identifying physicians who will be excellent members of the executive/physician leadership team is to note those doctors, young or old, who are straining at the tether to give you well-reasoned, articulately stated suggestions. It is well worth it to spend time and money offering such individuals opportunities to develop organizational leadership skills. This doesn't mean just taking or sending physicians off to "leadership seminars." It may mean that, but, more important, it means acting as a mentor to help interested physicians develop practical organizational leadership skills "on the job," as it were, in the process of participating in leadership activities.

The characteristics of a physician who will probably make a good leader are no different from the characteristics of an executive who makes a good leader instead of being satisfied with being just a manager. Some of these characteristics are summarized in table 2, page 48.

Discussion Points

1. In your organization, what characteristics do you value in members of the management team? In members of the leadership team?

2. In your organization, besides being concerned with identifying and developing physician leaders just to comply with external requirements for physician leadership, what efforts do you make to identify physicians interested in becoming physician leaders? What characteristics of these individuals cause you to identify them as potential leaders?

3. In your organization, what opportunities do you give interested physicians to develop their leadership skills?

4. In the course of meetings and projects, are you aware of opportunities to help physicians be better members of the leadership team? Should you be? Or should you leave development of physician leaders to underlings?

5. In your organization, what are three examples of recent issues, meetings, or projects in which participation of knowledgeable physician leaders with the characteristics listed in this chapter were helpful?

6. What are three examples of recent issues, meetings, or projects in which participation of knowledgeable physician leaders with the characteristics listed in this chapter could have been helpful but was not provided? Why was this shared leadership not provided?

References

1. Wills, G. *Certain Trumpets: The Nature of Leadership.* New York, N.Y.: Simon and Schuster, 1994, p. 17.

2. Thompson, R. *The Medical Staff Leader's Practical Guidebook.* Marblehead, Mass.: Opus, 1996, pp. 2-3.

Table 1. Some Differences between Leaders and Managers

CHARACTERISTIC	LEADER	MANAGER
Good With Details	Usually not. Prefers to deal with the big picture.	Yes. But must keep the big picture in view.
Integrity	Promises are kept. Positions of authority are not abused. Ethical values are important.	Nothing is wrong with telling one person one thing, and another person another. Ethical values are a distraction, not a key to success.
Vision	Knows the value of vision. Keeps people positioned to react to change. Plans, even though the future is uncertain.	Tomorrow's uncertain anyway, so why think about it. When promoted to executive, brings this view with him or her.
Sensitivity	Makes tough decisions when necessary, but not without considering and acknowledging their unwelcome impact on people.	Usually attempts to ride roughshod over other's feelings and concerns.
Analytical Skills	Questions assumptions. Figures out where opposition to plans is coming from, and why. Quickly sees flaws in newly implemented methods, and suggests changes.	Has little interest in asking, "Why?" Analysis is a waste of time. Just wants to know, "How?" "Tell me what to do and I'll get on with it."
Communication Skills	Thinks carefully about definitions and word choices. Suggestions to people are helpful suggestions, not personal attacks.	Sarcastically criticizes "jargon," yet buys into it! "Suggestions" to others are often personal attacks rather than helpful discussions.
Problem-Solving Behavior	Questions whether or not the problem is stated accurately. Shares information. Finds or develops several feasible ways to solve the problem.	Accepts statement of the problem as presented. Wants to keep information about the problem secret, even from others within the organization who could help in solving the problem! Seeks instant solutions.
Enjoys Being a "Mentor"	Likes helping people develop personally and professionally.	Views development in others as a threat to his or her own position and interests.
Can Lead Without Occupying a Position of Authority	Knows that "authority," "control," and "influence" are not synonyms. Leads whether or not in an official leadership position.	An ineffective leader, even if the person occupies a position with decision-making authority.
Has a Sense of Humor	Never takes him- or herself or any situation too seriously. But avoids being flippant.	Humor is not appreciated. It interferes with the job to be done.
Idea of "Being in Business"	Understands the idea of business as a fair exchange of goods and services, using money to avoid a total barter economy, with reasonable profit an expected result.	Believes the idea of "being in business" is to "make money." Any means justifies that end ("whatever it takes.")

Table 2. Some Characteristics of a True Leader*

• Integrity	The true leader's word can be respected. Promises are kept. Positions of authority are not abused in the interest of personal gain.
• Vision	Long-range goals are perceived as important, and uncertainty of the future is not used as an excuse to avoid planning and goal-setting.
• Sensitivity	True leaders not only listen to spoken words but also are alert for what is not being said and why.
• Analytical skills	Why aren't plans working out? Whose feelings are in the way? Which implementation methods have been chosen that will not achieve the anticipated objective? What are the right questions that must be asked and answered? The true leader will figure those things out.
• Communication skills	The true leader thinks carefully about word choices, in both written and oral communication. Communications are never intimidating, provoking, or angry, nor are they personal attacks.
• Problem-solving behavior	Unlike the leader of a political group, the organizational leader is a problem-solver, not a position-taker. For example, he or she favors sharing information, (within reason) so that informed, mutually beneficial decisions can be made.
• Enjoys "people projects"	The term "mentor" is an accolade often sought after by a true leader, who enjoys identifying and developing the best in others.
• Can lead whether or not in a position of authority	The true leader knows that authority, influence, persuasion, and control are not synonyms. Rather, the true leader depends on personal skills and attributes to influence the thinking and actions of people and to mold organizational culture.
• Sense of humor	The true leader never takes himself or herself too seriously. Often, without being flippant, the true leader relieves tense situations with appropriate humor. (Abraham Lincoln's style is a good example.)

*Reprinted with permission from Thompson, R., and Cofer, J. *Medical Staff Leader's Practical Guide*, third edition, Marblehead, MA.: Opus Communications, 1996

Chapter 8

Ten Keys to Establishing the True Partnership

Executives and physicians have at least one thing in common. Like most people, they prefer to stick with the 3 Cs, choosing only those options that are conventional, comfortable, and convenient.

Because of recent changes in the U.S. health care system, neither executives nor physicians can afford that approach.

There is no quick-and-easy, fool-proof, off-the-shelf, easy-installation plan for successfully working with physicians to share leadership in health care systems. Rather, the reader must apply his or her own management style and a unique blend of personal characteristics to the specific physician mix in his or her organization and community. However...

Neglecting one or any combination of the following 10 points is as close as there is to an easy, off-the-shelf method for *dooming* efforts at collaboration to a failure that can generate deep-seated and long-lasting conflicts.

1. Recruit Leaders Carefully

Some physicians respond well to the opportunity to be organizational leaders and some don't. To a great extent, the management team has the opportunity to carefully match specific leadership opportunities with the right physicians (see Chapter 9).

The "right physician" means a physician with interests, temperament, and availability that fit the needs of the organizational leadership opportunity, plus a reputation for objectivity and fairness. In addition, the "right" physician must either exhibit, or be willing to make the effort to develop, relevant organizational leadership skills.

Some physician readers will object to the notion that physician leaders are selected by anyone except the medical staff. That's because, in the old "organized hospital medical staff" model, CEOs were forced to work with "leaders" elected by popular vote of the medical staff. So the choice of "physician leaders" was political, or physicians just "rotated through," as opposed to physicians with organizational leadership skills being chosen. But in today's integrated delivery systems, that old-fashioned medical staff model has little relevance, except insofar as politically active physicians cling to remnants of it in the hospital component of the integrated system and insist that it still be included in Joint Commission requirements.[1]

Don't Over-Generalize, But...

Health care executives who successfully implement shared leadership learn to recognize, and deal differently with, the following types of physicians:

Dr. Wonderful: A sense of responsibility, a sense of humor without flippancy, clinical skills, interpersonal skills, a sense of fairness, analytical skills, and good communication skills make this doctor a delightful person with whom to share leadership.

Dr. Today: This doctor may be reluctant to change (who isn't?) but has at least most of Dr. Wonderful's characteristics, including a good analytical mind and willingness to understand the realities of events beyond his or her immediate control. His or her good questions can be quite valuable in helping members of the executive staff sharpen their thinking. And, as the executive staff effectively responds to these questions, this physician's value to the leadership team increases both because of his or her own increased understanding, and because he or she tells colleagues that "they seem to be listening!"

Dr. Yesterday: This doctor has the Gloria Patri mentality. ("As it was in the Beginning, it is now and ever shall be.") He or she stubbornly insists on helping everybody understand the error of their ways. Usually, Dr. Yesterday is not a good choice to be an organizational leader.

Dr. Tomorrow: This doctor is an innovator with vision who happens to be a physician. Usually he or she has the enthusiasm of an enjoyable puppy. ("This can be computerized, can't it!?!") An excellent choice for some sorts of shared leadership.

Dr. Scientific: This physician is a good leader in efforts to advance the cause of clinical services of a highly technical and complex nature.

Dr. Entrepreneur: You are probably most comfortable with this type of physician, as long as he or she is working with you instead of setting up clinical services that compete with yours. This member of your leadership team may be a subspecialist in a high-revenue-producing clinical specialty or an economic partner of your organization in some business venture.

Dr. Quality: This physician is genuinely concerned that the organization deliver clinical services that are dependable from the viewpoint of patients, residents and clients, and their family members. Once recognized as a valuable member of the leadership team only at Joint Commission survey time, this individual is now recognized as a major asset in a market that, for whatever reasons, increasingly demands a balanced value equation

(Value = Cost Efficiency + Dependable Clinical Services, from the viewpoint of users (see also page 9).

Dr. Trouble: A few short years ago, this species of physician was ubiquitous. Now, while in no danger of extinction, the number of Dr. Troubles has significantly decreased. He or she is easily recognized. He or she usually has excellent oratorical skills and uses them to be an effective meeting bully. Urges physician colleagues to act independently as opposed to cooperating with "the enemy," seen to be health care executives, attorneys, some nurses, and sometimes just about everybody with whom he or she comes in contact. Definitely not a candidate to be an organizational leader. (Amazingly, conversion of this physician type to a Dr. Today is sometimes possible.)

Dr. Litigator: This physician may be working on, or have obtained, a law degree. He or she begins most sentences with, "On the advice of legal counsel." Handle with care. May be a great adversarial political leader but usually does not possess the characteristics necessary to be a good organizational leader.

2. Succinctly Summarize a Shared Practical Ethic and Use This Document as an Operational Guideline

Virtually all providers' mission statements and marketing literature proclaim their organizations to be delivering the highest quality of care. However, they invariably fail to specify the measures of quality that purchasers and patients could interpret and use for provider selection.[2]

No matter how eloquent, mission statements and values/ethics statements are seldom used in operational meetings of some managed care organizations. Individuals who do not share a common practical ethic will never achieve the true shared leadership state that is critical to success in the next phases of managed care.[3] For a detailed discussion of this point, see chapter 6.

3. Be as Available as You Are to Another Executive

When a physician calls another physician, the call is put right through. And when a physician calls an organizational executive, he or she is told, "He's in a meeting, but he might have time to call you back either today or tomorrow."

It's true, an executive's life is one meeting after another. And a good secretary knows how to screen phone calls to preserve desk-work time, and is often instructed to do so. That's fine.

In fact, it's necessary. Everybody wants to talk to the head honcho. But it's possible to protect your time and privacy in ways that offend only the unreasonable. For example, get yourself one of those office wall signs that says, "I'll talk to anyone about anything, but not just anytime."

With respect to physicians, it's only necessary to use the same phone-answering policy for physician leaders that you use for senior executives. And don't forget to so instruct your secretary. By the way, some grass-roots clinicians will accuse you of cronyism and try to force you to extend "open anytime" availability to every single physician on the medical staff or physician panel. Just say no.

If you offer the privilege of reasonably easy availability to physician leaders and one physician leader abuses the privilege, he or she (but not every physician leader) should lose the privilege. Chances are his or her colleagues will understand and (silently) applaud.

By the way, the same telephone-answering scenario exists in a doctor's office. Front office personnel are good at screening calls. When an executive telephones a physician, she won't be told "he's in a meeting," but she may be told, "He's with a patient." Well, when I was in pediatric practice and Mary Jane would tell someone, "He's with a patient," sometimes I was with a patient and sometimes I was at my desk completing records of office visits and going through the day's mail. So be sure to explain to physician leaders that you expect the same telephone availability privilege that you extend to them. And they should so instruct their front office personnel.

4. Help the Physician Understand and Accept Today's Realities

Physicians *know* what's going on in health care, but knowledge is two steps removed from influencing changes in behavior. Behavior change is only motivated by *understanding* and *accepting* what is known.

A key task is to help physicians understand and accept that, so far, there is only one clear consequence of the Great Health Care Reform Debate of 1993-1994.

Health care dollars will never again flow easily to separatists.

Once this is understood by both physicians and executives, shared leadership usually follows.

5. Listen. Really Hear What Physicians Say

A common physician complaint over the years has been, "Administration invites us to a meeting or a retreat saying they value our input in their plans and decisions, but, when they get us there, they just lecture to us about why we should support what's already been decided."

If that were just interesting history, it wouldn't be very important. But I was surprised to hear the same thing as recently as 1998, from a group of hand-selected physicians, in a meeting of a health care system's medical advisory group!

Not only is it polite and politic to listen to reasonable and articulate physicians; sometimes it is a major key to avoiding costly mistakes in planning, including inaccurate financial projections.

6. Learn What a Doctor Does When He or She Is Doctoring

Uncle Abner said that the person who has took a bull by the tail has learnt sixty or seventy times as much as a person who hasn't.—*Tom Sawyer Abroad,* Mark Twain.

If I were asked to suggest the two most potentially helpful points in this book, I would select this point and all of Chapter 6.

Ever since Medicare and Medicaid, and with greater intensity since DRG payment and then managed care, "working with physicians" has been primarily a matter of urging doctors to understand the executive's world. That is, we push physicians to understand and accept the realities of how organizations work and how they can help us. Many physicians have responded by becoming much more sophisticated about organizational matters.

Now, in the era of truly shared leadership, successful executives should return the favor. That is, better understand the frustrations and fears of clinical practice and its awesome one-on-one responsibilities. The positive impact on the executive/physician working relationship can be immediate and sometimes dramatic.

For example, "risk management" to executives means reducing legal liability. Concern is for the organization, because (so far) malpractice judgments against health care executives are unheard of. But here's a different perspective on the meaning of "risk:"

The first lumbar puncture ("spinal tap") I did was as a medical student, under the supervision of a resident-in-training. With the hesitation of the novice, I positioned the patient on his side with knees drawn up under his chin, opened the procedure tray, prepared the needle and specimen tubes, put on rubber gloves (ruining the first pair in my anxiety), and administered the local anesthetic.

Murmuring reassurances and brief explanations to the patient, I selected the correct intervertebral interspace and gingerly inserted the needle. And then from the needle came dripping...you may applaud...clear spinal fluid! Well, sure, that's a big deal, because a "bloody tap" is not an uncommon occurrence. It then took me several minutes to let fluid drip into the specimen tubes, label the tubes, withdraw the needle, and cover the small hole in the patient's back with a bandaid. I was feeling pretty good, let me tell you. Now I was finished, except to be sure I had not damaged a nerve root. "Wiggle your toes, please," I instructed the patient. Nothing happened. In a louder voice I repeated, "Please wiggle your toes." The patient said, "I can't."

The seasoned resident remained calm. But I was panic-stricken! After we left the patient in post-tap position (flat on his back), the resident quietly advised me to go have a cup of coffee and re-examine the patient in about an hour. I still remember that hour as one of the longest in my life. I wasn't worried about being sued. I didn't know anything about malpractice then. I was figuring, "What am I going to do instead of get an MD degree after they kick me out of medical school!?"

Finally the hour was up. Dejectedly, I returned to the patient's room. The patient was lying on his back as instructed, in good humor, having no pain or discomfort, and could now wiggle his toes and move his legs normally!

I reported happily to my resident physician supervisor and asked him what happened. He could barely keep from laughing as he told me, "Thompson, you did the tap fine but naturally, since it was your first one, pretty slow. Next time you have 40 minutes to spare, lie down on your side with your feet doubled up under your chin and see if your feet don't go to sleep."

Little wonder, then, that physicians find it laughable when one interpretation of "risk" is a plea by a middle manager to "please come to my risk management committee meeting and support my risk management program."

It may be impossible to fully understand the logic of statements and stances of surgeons on issues related to both patient care and budget concerns until one has visited the O.R. while an operation is in progress and come out with bloodstains on one's shoe covers.

Dealing with the realities of clinical practice can cause physicians to engage in some organizational behavior that looks pretty silly, unless and until the roots of the behavior are understood. For example, a physician must often be vigorously decisive in the face of incomplete information, such as choosing and starting antibiotics before culture results are back. This makes physicians famous for being intuitionists. That means that their "contribution" in a meeting may be, "We're wasting time and money here. We don't need data, consultants, or financial projections. Let's just move ahead."

Without a clear understanding of the roots of such behavior, the working relationship can be strained to the point of counterproductive conflicts, such as by the executive's decision to "avoid this hassle" by excluding physicians from the decision-making process.

The following is a very serious suggestion. Ask two or three physician leaders if you may observe them at work for an hour or two. Or, at the very least, plan to spend 15 minutes in one clinical care area or another once or twice a week and observe the hustle and bustle.

If you don't like that suggestion, you're lucky that I'm not one of your doctors. When I was "Chief of Pediatrics" (a physician leader), I would occasionally hound Bruce (the CEO) or Jim (the COO) until one or the other would come up to the Pediatric Intensive Care Unit with me for a cup of coffee...and so I could show them a patient or two I wanted them to see.

We were all very busy people. So they pretty much knew that I had an agenda, which was usually to bolster my case for needed staff, space, or equipment. But they came anyway.

In fact, we developed a good relationship. I became enough of an executive insider that Bruce occasionally responded to a written request from me in a way that saved a lot of time. I would just get the request back, stamped with Bruce's famous "This Is Bull" stamp.

As a result of this sometimes reluctant collaboration, our pediatric services turned into a good "leader," providing a good public image for the medical center, which was better marketing than programs for which we could have paid a lot of money.

7. Share Relevant Information, within Reason

Sharing leadership requires sharing information. That isn't what we're conditioned to do. In recent years, health care has been characterized as much by legal, financial, and political

manipulation as by a direct interest in clinical care. And in the legal, financial, and political arenas, the paradigm is secrecy. So (we think) we are better at keeping secrets than at sharing information.

One thought that may help us decide to share information to a reasonable degree is that, often, "confidentiality" is only a myth in which we choose to believe.

Implement a policy of a reasonable degree of sharing information with physicians. (The qualifier is necessary, because some physicians, ideally not selected as having organizational leadership characteristics, want to know everything, including such matters as the details of the CEO's contract. Tell the physicians, "That's board business.")

Of course, some matters must be kept confidential. But the degree to which we practice "confidentiality" reached a ridiculous extreme in the overly adversarial era of the 1980s and early 1990s.

Example

The author conducted a leadership training seminar in which several physicians became interested in new, positive methods of drawing conclusions about physician performance from relevant data. This interest was undoubtedly whetted by a well-respected doctor who is president of a physician group successful in landing contracts with managed care organizations. This person advised the group, "This stuff isn't just for the Joint Commission anymore. We'll be using these kind of data to pick doctors for our practice group and to decide which ones to keep."

The group was discouraged, however, because they did not believe that data such as those demonstrated were locally available, and they believed that setting up such a system would be costly and impractical.

After the seminar, the CEO asked the VPMA and me to come into her office for a moment. After swearing us to secrecy, she showed us a collection of data of which she is justifiably quite proud. These data are made available only to the Finance Committee of the Board (on which there are no physicians). And some of these good data produced by this locally developed system are exactly what physician leaders need to proceed with learning the new positive methods of evaluating physician performance, which can be of great benefit to the system as well as to physicians and to users of clinical services.

8. Help Physician Leaders Understand How to "Argue"

"Argue" and "quarrel" are not synonyms.

Learning to argue productively means three things:

First, productive argument means learning that arguing in the sense of quarreling is hardly ever productive. Quarrelsome individuals are often good at controlling meetings by effective use of three strategies, which are to provoke, intimidate, and distract other members of the group. Unfortunately, two of the best places to observe these meeting bullies at work are meetings of Florida condominium associations and meetings of a "general medical staff."

Orient physician leaders to some simple, informal rules of courtesy in debate. For example, Thompson's (unpublished) Rules of Order include:

- Only one person should speak at a time.

- Address your comments to the chair, not to each other. (This makes it harder for meeting bullies to operate.)

- Nobody speaks twice until everybody who wants to has spoken once.

- Plan your remarks. Make your point in three minutes or less.

- If Roberts' Rules of Order ever become the focus of discussion, we are making the common mistake of discussing procedure instead of substance.

Second, learning to argue productively means learning not to argue at all if there is no substantive disagreement. The key to avoiding arguments when two people don't really disagree is careful definition of terms. For example, two people arguing heatedly about the use of revenue from "hospital operations" should first be sure they are talking about the same thing. Believe it or not, I have facilitated discussions in which executives were using this term in the usual management sense, but it turned out that one or two physicians in the group thought the discussion was about revenue generated for the hospital as a result of surgeons performing surgical procedures in the operating suite!

And, in discussing nursing needs, what does "dedicated nurse" mean? To a physician, it is most likely to mean a nurse who is committed to meeting the needs of patients. But it can also mean a nurse who does not "float," but works in only one clinical area.

Finally, arguing effectively means knowing when the argument (debate) is over. That is, following the divergent phase of decision making, which is listing and debating all possible options, comes the convergent phase of deciding (by consensus or by vote) which option to implement. Once that decision is made, the time to argue (even in the positive sense) is over. Now it is time for members of the shared leadership team to pull together to implement the chosen option effectively, so that the desired result is achieved.

9. Go Back to Square One

A *good* leader is always willing to revisit an issue to see if new happenings necessitate, or make possible, new and better approaches to an old issue. A very good leader has an uncanny sense of timing, knowing the right moment to reconsider a matter for which a former decision or solution is no longer feasible, adequate, or relevant. And an *excellent* leader may actually plan to discuss an issue periodically as a matter of strategy.

I characterize willingness to revisit an issue as excellent leadership because I do it myself. And so do you. Don't you often figure that it will be necessary to present an item to the board three times before obtaining its approval? The first time will be an "information only" presentation. The second time will be a "first reading," and the third time the item will appear on the board agenda as a (now familiar) "Action Item."

On the national level, I won't be surprised if providers someday participate in a joint public/private effort to go back to square one and reconsider current national health care policy. That is, a policy-setting commission may someday consider available options so far ignored for building a unique U.S. health care system that blends the best of the competitive model with single-payer efficiencies.[4]

10. Help Physicians Find Their Organizational Niches.

Help physicians discover organizational roles in which they can feel the satisfaction of truly contributing to the organization's success. ("Contributing" in this context means contributing ideas and responsible accomplishment of necessary tasks, not money contributions.) There can be no better example of a win-win or value-added situation in any business.

To find his or her niche, the physician must understand both how organizations work and his or her own needs and motivations. For a detailed discussion of this point, see the book that is intended as a companion to this one.[5]

Discussion Points

1. Reread the section headings in this chapter. Which of these 10 points would you modify in some way? Which would you delete from the list? What additional points would you add to this list?

2. In your organization, are physician leaders treated with respect, including showing respect by arguing with them (in a productive way) when necessary? Or is your attitude toward physician leaders condescending or servile? What approach is best?

3. Dr. Wonderful and Dr. Today have been placed on a committee with Dr. Yesterday for the specific purpose of "getting Dr. Yesterday to see the light." Is this a wise and productive strategy? Why or why not?

4. In your organization, how often is the mission statement or values/ethics statement available in operational meetings and referred to as a guideline?

5. Think of a physician you respect as a clinician and as a person. How would he or she respond if you asked to watch him or her work? If you haven't asked, how do you know that would be the response?

6. In your organization, what information do you share with physician leaders? Should any of that information be withheld? Should you add any information items to the list of what is shared with physician leaders?

References

1. Thompson, R. *Compliance Guide to the Joint Commission's Medical Staff Standards.* Marblehead, Mass.: Opus, 1998.

2. Mohlenbrock, W. "The Physician Imperative: Define, Measure, and Improve Health Care Quality. *Physician Executive* 24(3):47-54, May-June 1998.

3. Coile, R. *The Five Stages of Managed Care: Strategies for Providers, HMOs, and Suppliers.* Chicago, Ill.: Health Administration Press, 1997.

4. Thompson, R. "Sustainability as the Linchpin of Public Policy and Industry Initiatives." *Physician Executive* 24(4):52-5, July-Aug. 1998.

5. Thompson, R. *So You've Been Integrated, Now What? Opportunities for Physicians Practicing in Managed Care Settings.* Tampa, Fla.: American College of Physician Executives, 1996, p. 15.

Chapter 9

Physician Members of the Leadership Team: Who's in Charge of What?

A "leadership team" is a group of individuals with defined high-level responsibilities and the authority to work with others to carry out these responsibilities. Members of a leadership team, looking at both the short-term and long-range view, together create and implement a shared ethic and mutually acceptable strategies to achieve common goals.

The senior leadership team of an integrated system and its component parts is made up of executives, senior managers, physician leaders, board members, and frontline clinical practitioners.

A major key to success of this leadership team is matching the unique personality characteristics, interests, and skills of physician members of the leadership team to organizational roles, work assignments, and responsibilities. Here are some examples.

Sharing Leadership with the Physician Entrepreneur

The physician entrepreneur can be an extremely valuable ally of the integrated system because of his or her vision of a lucrative community medical service and how it might be established and funded. But a physician entrepreneur may also be a troublesome thorn in the organization's side, because he or she successfully sets up clinical services that compete with some of those offered by the organization.

The difference is often a matter of how well the organization's executive staff understands and implements the concept of shared leadership, which implies some degree of flexibility.

Example

In one community, Dr. Osseus, head of a prominent orthopedic group, approached senior management of the MediBest Health System with an offer to move his base of operations (no pun intended) to MediBest's central campus. Negotiations began. When negotiations faltered, it was not over the issue of how to divide profits. Rather, as is often the case when dealing with physicians, potential deal-breakers were the definition of control, where the venture should be housed (the CEO wanted to make over existing space; the orthopedist

wanted a new building), and how much new equipment should be purchased and who should pay for it.

The CEO of the organization gambled and lost. He knew that his system was the only game in town, which he defined as being the only system in town, so he figured that the orthopedist was in a weak bargaining position.

The CEO stated a position and refused to budge. He was totally inflexible, refusing even to consider some compromise solutions suggested by the orthopedist in the two areas most important to the orthopedist.

As a result, the orthopedist developed his own group of investors (some physicians and some executives of local industries with more vision than that of the health care organization's CEO). The Osseus Regional Bone and Joint Center was created and today is an independent orthopedic center that draws referrals from miles around and is a huge financial success.

In another community, an entrepreneurial orthopedist's offer to become part of the system was handled differently. The CEO worked with the entrepreneurial physician to arrive at reasonable compromises on issues important to the orthopedist, because he understands the unique point of view of an entrepreneurial physician who is also a frontline clinician! In this community, the resulting orthopedic center is now a major revenue-producer, image-builder, and marketing tool that benefits all components of the integrated system.

A Caveat

Some health care organizations, particularly their hospital components, have caused problems for themselves by being too eager to bring in an entrepreneurial physician to "capture a market niche." The central theme of these scenarios is hasty credentialing, resulting in unnecessary and expensive legal hassles.

Sharing Leadership with Physician Leaders of "the Organized Medical Staff" in the Hospital/Medical Center Component of the Integrated Delivery System

Increasingly, system executives realize that the hospital component of the integrated system is either the jewel in the system's crown, or the system's Achilles' heel.

The hospital (or "medical center") component of a system will always be the most critical focus of public applause or public criticism of the system. The hospital will always be a

major determinant of whether the bottom line is red or black and a huge key to satisfactory compliance with state regulations and Joint Commission requirements. And even if life in these United States ever becomes less aggressive and litigious (a development that is not yet in any futurist's predictions) and even as inpatient care becomes less necessary, the hospital will remain the source of our most troublesome and often most preventable legal tangles.

Across the economy, power is shifting from producers to consumers. Yet health care continues to act out producer-dominant behaviors, and this is setting the stage for trouble ahead.[1]

The acute care component of any system has this high-priority position because illness and injury are events that sooner or later interrupt and threaten the life-styles of every U.S. citizen except those who die suddenly.

In spite of complex medical technology, and in spite of "managed care," the mortality rate in this country remains the same. It's one apiece. You'll get yours.

Thus, while the future is undeniably here, in the sense of offering wellness services and of focusing on systems improvement, some of the past is still with us and will accompany us into the new millennium.

Here are some examples of working with physician leaders in hospitals, which often means understanding and dealing with an old medical staff organizational structure better suited to the simpler hospitals of 80 years ago, which is when this structure was created.[2] For further details, see resources that specifically focus on shared leadership activities in the hospital setting[3,4]

The Vice President for Medical Affairs (VPMA)

The VPMA is an individual with an MD or a DO degree whose interests and aptitudes have led him or her to prefer organizational work to daily care of patients.

The days when a VPMA might also have been a frontline clinician are behind us.

The first VPMAs (medical directors) in hospitals retained a clinical practice. One reason for this is that the first VPMA in many settings was chosen from among physicians practicing in the community. The nature of the position then (just a few years ago) was that it could be filled by a successful and respected physician ready for semi-retirement. There was no reason the VPMA should not have time to retain his or her practice, or a portion of it.

Besides, even though acceptance of VPMA's by frontline clinicians was slow, it was sped up a little bit by the comfort that frontline clinicians could have in dealing with one of their well-known and clinically respected colleagues.

Today, the combination of clinical, entrepreneurial, management, compliance, public relations, and ambassadorial responsibilities of a VPMA in the hospital component of the integrated system leaves no time for practice. But the wise VPMA takes pains to reassure frontline clinicians that he or she values and understands their perspective.

The VPMA should not be referred to as a "physician." Frontline clinicians prefer that this term be used to refer to people holding MD or DO degrees who actually diagnose, treat, and operate on patients. Actually, observing this definition of physician serves a useful purpose. For years, executives have tried to sell medical staffs on projected plans, purchases, mergers, and expansions by claiming "physician input" to the project. Frontline physicians privately scoffed at this claim, knowing that the "physician" providing the input was an MD-MBA who might or might not have finished a specialty residency and who had never cared for patients.

One might expect someone with the title of vice president for medical affairs to be a senior executive with line authority. From the executive's view, he or she is. However, with respect to the medical staff in a hospital, the VPMA is often still a staff position with little or no direct authority over the hospital's physicians. At best, the VPMA in today's hospitals shares executive authority with both an elected medical staff president (or "chief of staff") and a medical executive committee whose members may still be selected by popular vote.

The Medical Executive Function

Practicing physicians who accept a position on the medical executive committee must be oriented to the committee's relationship to other hospital executives and to the governing board. This is a task that cannot be delegated to middle management. The CEO should take the lead and should be assisted by the VPMA, the vice president for nursing services, the VP for finance, and the board chair.

Only a few organizations entrust the executive function to a committee rather than to an individual. In fact, only two examples come immediately to mind—hospital medical staffs and Florida condominium associations. In neither case does the model work very well.

A single executive, or a three- or four-member medical executive cabinet, would be better able to make and execute decisions and plans in a timely manner than a 10-or 15-member medical executive committee. So why do some physicians still resist adopting this sound organizational principle?

One reason is that the agenda and the proceedings of many medical executive committees are still more like the agenda of a medical legislative committee. A key to helping physicians learn the difference between the executive function in organizations, the legislative function in government, and political activities such as those of a medical society is to put a definition of "The Executive Function in Organizations" into the medical staff bylaws.[5]

Another reason small executive groups are still opposed by many physicians is lack of training in and experience with commonly used organizational procedures. For example, many physicians still believe that the medical executive committee must be "collegial" and do not understand the concept of a small executive group that obtains input prior to meetings by such mechanisms as phone interviews and questionnaires. Plus, the small executive group can always ask key individuals to serve as specific resources on a specific agenda issue.[6]

The central issue is (lack of) trust. This is the same problem that was encountered during the U.S. Constitutional Convention in 1787.

"At once Wilson moved that the executive consist of a single person. A considerable pause ensued. It was hard for any of the delegates to think of a single executive without thinking of a king, and George III had become the symbol of the rule that Americans had thrown off. The debate went over to Monday, June 4 (1787). Finally it was decided that if there should be three heads in the national executive, then there could be neither vigor nor tranquility."[7]

Some physicians have great difficulty thinking of a single executive without thinking of a king. And the dictatorial management style of some CEOs in the 1980s and early 1990s, before the continuous quality improvement (CQI) management style, with its emphasis on empowerment, became the norm, did not help physicians accept the "executive" concept.

Chairs of Clinical Departments of the Medical Staff

In the context of working with physicians, many organizational tasks can be accomplished effectively only by an individual with a unique combination of five characteristics—relevant authority, respect of most co-workers, a reputation for objectivity and fairness, relevant clinical expertise, and status as a "colleague" or "true peer." No one in the organizational structure combines all five of these qualities except a relevant and responsible physician leader, such as the chair of a clinical department of the medical staff.

Physicians Who Are Credentialing Specialists

The most familiar example of executive/physician leader shared leadership is credentialing and privileging independent clinical practitioners (ICPs), including physicians.

Until World War I, U.S. doctors had a unique relationship with the "superintendents" of local "community hospitals." Physicians enjoyed complete freedom to make up the treatments of patients as they went along and to perform any operations they chose to perform, whether or not they had done them before or had even seen them done. (To this day, a popular maxim in medical education is "See one, do one, teach one.")

Then, in 1919, the American College of Surgeons (ACS) responded to two separate but related studies[8,9] indicating that current training and practice habits of U.S. physicians were inconsistent, to say the least, and that better patient results might be achieved by changes in medical education and by some standardization of medical practice in U.S. hospitals. ACS framed and implemented a five-point "Minimum Standard" for U.S. hospitals[2] and accredited hospitals that met this standard. (This was the origin of the organization we know today as JCAHO.)

Point 2 in the original ACS Minimum Standard was "that membership upon the staff be restricted to physicians and surgeons who are (a) full graduates of medicine in good standing and legally licensed to practice in their respective states and provinces, (b) competent in their respective fields, and (c) worthy in character."[2]

That was the beginning of what we know today as "credentialing and privileging."

Note that, because ACS was responding to concerns about the nature of medical training and the consistency of patient care in U.S. hospitals, it is quite likely that the predominant original purpose of credentialing was to improve the consistency of medical care services available to patients. That's important to note, because executives and managers who have entered the field in the past 20 years may have the mistaken impression that

credentialing physicians is just an organizational power tool used to carve out big chunks of "market share."

Executives need the help of physician leaders to work through several evolving issues in credentialing and privileging that can be summarized as a rediscovery of the patient-protective purpose of credentialing physicians and other licensed independent practitioners.

The most important development in credentialing and privileging is a trend away from a compulsively prescriptive approach fostered by the notion that each and every "credentialing criterion" is a stand-alone, absolute legal standard. The trend is toward a more descriptive approach that features a variety of information sources (licensure, formal training, recent clinical experience, newly available formats of valid performance data, etc.) combined to form the basis of action on a physician's application for clinical privileges.

The old legalistic prescriptive approach resulted in credentialing and privileging activities characterized primarily by legal maneuvering. The new approach of using several credentialing guidelines together to frame a recommendation on an application relates credentialing to professionalism as originally intended.

Some traditionally thinking executives and attorneys may at first be dismayed by this development. That's to be expected, because we have become so conditioned to thinking of credentialing and privileging as a legal and economic issue. It will take some time for us to fully appreciate the value to our organization, including its physicians, of truly patient-protective credentialing and privileging. That benefit will come in recognizable forms, such as a good public image, avoidance of unnecessary legal problems related to care by undependable practitioners, and success in demonstrating full value (reasonable cost plus dependable medical services) to contractors.

For those interested in more details, see available resources that contain practical examples of new forms, letters, guidelines, and other tools used in today's modern credentialing and privileging activities.[3,4,10-14]

Physicians with Topical Specialties

Physicians with a professional interest in such topics as infectious diseases and infection control, use of blood and blood products, pharmacy and therapeutics, or subspecialty areas such as various surgical subspecialties can be extremely valuable to the physician/executive leadership team.

One example is the usefulness of these individuals as advisors to department chairs, the medical executive committee, and other relevant officials who must frame and use valid conclusions from data reflecting physician performance and patient outcomes. That is, the responsible chair of internal medicine may practice in the subspecialty of endocrinology. So he may appoint a "physician analyst" with clinical expertise in hematology to help him review and draw conclusions from data about how dependably members of the department of medicine are ordering blood and blood products.

Hospital-Level Medical Advisory Group

A group of physician advisors who currently engage in clinical practice should be invited to meet periodically with hospital executives and physician leaders for the purpose of "brainstorming" about issues of importance to frontline clinicians. Members of this group may or may not currently hold official leadership positions. Name this group something other than a "Committee," because it is not the committee meeting mentality we are looking for here.

The cross-communication function being described here is not a medical executive committee agenda item. The medical executive committee meeting is a business meeting with information items and action items. The medical advisory group may or may not have a specific agenda, and it never votes, because it has no official authority.

Physicians invited to participate on the medical advisory group are carefully selected by the executive/physician leadership team. Criteria should include respected clinical skills, good communication skills, a reputation for objectivity and fairness, and a high degree of clinical activity in the hospital. A cross-section of medical specialties should be included, and hospital-based physicians must not be over-represented.

The medical advisory group should not be overly concerned with regularity of meetings, formal meeting procedures, or "development of minutes." In addition to regular short (one-hour) monthly meetings, members of the medical advisory group should be on call to the executive staff and physician leaders to discuss issues that may arise related to specific clinical practice areas.

The benefits and the effectiveness of the medical advisory group are measured by the degree to which members' participation increases the network of physician support for plans and activities related to physicians' practices.

The leaders of the medical advisory group should be guided, in such matters as deciding which issues to discuss, by a policy that lists issues that affect physician's practices. An example of such a policy, for use by both the hospital-level medical advisory group and the system-level medical advisory group, is shown in figure 1, page 73.

Sharing Leadership with Physicians at the Network/System Level

System VPMA

Some integrated systems have a VPMA at the system level and some don't. When the position of VPMA was first created at both the hospital and system levels, one stated purpose of the position was to build bridges. That is, it was expected that this person would contribute greatly to the evolution of shared leadership between executives and physicians. And, at first, this is exactly what happened.[15]

I dug out some notes about the position of corporate VPMA that I made in May 1993. I see from my notes that I had telephoned ACPE and five corporate VPMAs and, from that input, had drafted a "Sample Position Description for a Corporate or System VPMA" at the request of a system CEO That 1993 draft, with some updated language, is reproduced as figure 2, page 76. You can see that I expected the position of VPMA to continue evolving in the direction of relating very closely to the goal of developing shared leadership between the executive staff and the medical staff.

Boy, was I wrong!

Today's system level VPMA, reflecting priorities in the current profit-taking health care policy model, is commonly expected to focus on managed care contracting, insurance issues, entrepreneurial innovations, networking with other health care agencies, untangling legal messes, and community public relations. Obviously, this leaves little time and energy for focusing on shared leadership issues. One exception is that, when a system has a VPMA, he or she usually staffs a systemwide medical advisory group.

Today's search firms and sophisticated VPMAs, with their MBA-degrees, can get a good laugh out of my old 1993 "sample job description" draft and out of how wrong I was. Yet events of recent years make me wonder if it might not be valuable to reintroduce into the mix some of the VPMA responsibilities included in people's 1993 thinking, so that physicians throughout a system might see clearly that there is a system-level interest in promoting shared leadership. For example, just look at the "Position Overview" in figure 2. Are system and managed care organization VPMAs today made to feel comfortable with being "the primary advocate ensuring that considerations of dependable clinical performance are included in executive/management decisions?" And on page 3 of figure 2, are most system VPMAs made available to "help local medical staff leaders communicate effectively with the board, the executive staff, and frontline clinicians at their own locations?"

In the appendix you will find at least three case studies in which the timely involvement of a system VPMA with a job description similar to that in figure 2 could have prevented these scenarios from being picked as unfortunate examples of the critical need for shared leadership.

At the very least, rewards of such an approach should include getting help from physician leaders that could help executives avoid future mistakes like some made in the past, including setting up modern-day fee-splitting arrangements with physicians and gagging frontline practitioners.

System Directors of Clinical Services
The organizational structure of some clinical service areas may include a systemwide medical director. Examples include pulmonology, rehabilitation medicine, cardiovascular services, women's health care services, etc. The duties of the MDs or DOs who are clinical directors of these areas include some combination of administrative and clinical responsibilities. The very specific clinical expertise of these individuals, their ordinarily aggressive work ethic, and the respect they usually enjoy among physicians make them very valuable members of the executive/physician leadership team.

Systemwide Medical Advisory Group
The system VPMA should staff a systemwide medical advisory group whose choice of discussion topics should be guided by a policy that lists issues that affect physician's practices. An example of such a policy, for use by both the hospital-level medical advisory group and the system-level medical advisory group, is shown in figure 1.

Physicians on the Board of Directors
Some physicians have the interests, aptitudes, analytical skills, and interpersonal skills to make great board members and some don't. The board must retain control of how all board members are selected, including physician members of the board.

A physician board member must adopt the broad perspective of any board member and must not use a seat on the board to champion the cause of any particular specialty, subspecialty, or practice group. An exception is that some boards invite physicians who hold formal positions of authority (such as a medical staff president) to participate in board meetings, sometimes as a member of the board. In that case, the individual is expected to serve on the board in his or her official capacity and thus is one valuable channel of "medical staff input."

Some executives may be slow to see the need for physicians on the board. That's understandable, because in most businesses the board of directors does not share decision making with frontline workers. Nobody suggests that every bank board include a teller, or that every symphony board include the principal cellist or even the concertmaster. But in health care, frontline practitioners have executive decision-making authority in the context of caring for each individual patient, client, resident, beneficiary, and member. Unless that fact is acknowledged and accepted at the board level, financial projections can be in error and even the best-laid organizational plans may fail.

Example

The executive staffs and boards of three (of seven) hospitals in one U.S. city decided to merge and form a small system to improve their competitive position in the community and in order to secure managed care contracts. Several physician leaders, usually known for their support of the hospitals, advised against this move, citing long-established physician referral patterns that followed different lines than the "centers of excellence" planned by the new system. The executives and board members dismissed these objections as simply the well-known opposition of physicians-as-a-whole to any sort of change, especially if there is a disturbance of local autonomy.

The merger proceeded and barely survived serious financial difficulties encountered in its first few years of existence. Financial projections were wrong. Anticipated revenues were not generated. The reason? Sure enough, outside consultants had generated figures using an assumption about cross-referrals between the three hospitals that was totally contrary to the long-established referral patterns of physicians practicing in the community, which continued within the context of managed care plans available in the city.

So physicians' participation in leadership in this instance turned out to be quite valuable. Or at least it could have been, had executives and board members carefully considered this input and questioned financial projections before the merger occurred.

Discussion Points

1. Think about the medical staff of your organization. Name two or three "entrepreneurial physicians." Name two or three with an interest in developing data to confirm dependable physician performance. Name two or three physicians who would be good members of the system's medical advisory group.

In your organization, are the interests and aptitudes of individual physicians correctly matched to organizational roles?

2. In the hospital component of your integrated system, how are frontline clinicians who are members of the organization's executive group (such as members of the medical executive committee) oriented to their relationship to other organizational executives?

3. In your organization, does the job description of a hospital VPMA and/or system VPMA contain any of the elements listed in figure 2? Should it? Why or why not? Do the duties of your VPMA(s) relate visibly and effectively to the development and maintenance of shared executive/physician leadership? Why or why not?

4. Are there physicians on your system board? If not, should there be? Why or why not? If so, how are physician members of the board chosen? How are they oriented so they can "wear the right hat" to system board meetings?

References

1. Sheehy, B., and others. *The Blind Spot*. La Jolla, Calif.: Governance Institute, 1998.

2. *Minimum Standard for Hospitals*. Chicago, Ill.: American College of Surgeons, 1919.

3. Thompson, R. *The Medical Staff Leader's Practical Guidebook*, Third Edition. Marblehead, Mass.: Opus Communications, 1996.

4. Thompson, R. *The Compliance Guide to the Medical Staff Standards*: Winning *Strategies For Your JCAHO Survey*, Second Edition. Marblehead, Mass.: Opus Communications, 1998.

5. *Medical Staff Portfolio*. Sample Medical Staff Bylaws, 4th Edition. Dunedin, Fla.: Thompson, Mohr and Associates, Inc., 1998.

6. *Medical Staff Portfolio*. Medical Executive Committee Guidelines, Policies, and Methods Manual. Dunedin, Fla.: Thompson, Mohr and Associates, Inc., 1996.

7. Van Doren, C. The Great Rehearsal: T*he Story of the Making and Ratifying of the Constitution of the United States*. New York, N.Y.: Penguin Books, 1986, p. 55.

8. Flexner, A. *Medical Education in the United States and Canada*. New York, N.Y.: Carnegie Foundation for the Advancement of Teaching, 1910.

9. Codman, E. "The Product of a Hospital." *Archives of Pathology and Laboratory Medicine* 114(11):1106-11, Nov. 1990.

10. *1998 Hospital Accreditation Standards* ("Pocket size" edition). MS.5.4.1, MS.5.4.2, MS.5.4.4, and MS.5.4.5, page 232. Oakbrook Terrace, Ill.: Joint Commission on Accreditation of Healthcare Organizations, 1998.

11. Various publications and educational programs. Marblehead, Mass.: Credentialing Resource Center.

12. Various publications and educational programs. Pittsburgh, Pa.: Credentialing Institute.

13. Various publications and educational programs. Tampa, Fla.: American College of Physician Executives.

14. *Medical Staff Portfolio*. Thompson, Mohr and Associates, Inc. Dunedin, FL. Thompson, Richard E., MD.

15. Thompson, R *Keys to Winning Physician Support*, First Edition. Tampa, Fla.: American College of Physician Executives, 1991, p. 39.

Figure 1. Sample Policy for Participation of Practicing Physicians in Decisions of Relevant Integrated Health Care Delivery Systems (IHCDS) Authorities that Affect the Delivery of Dependable Medical Care Services*

To be modified as necessary, then approved by the Governing Boards and Physician Leadership of all components of the IHCDS

This document does not require legal review. It is intended as an organizational guideline, not an absolute legal standard.

Selection of Participating Practicing Physicians

Practicing physicians are selected, ad hoc, to participate in management decisions affecting their areas of clinical practice.

Selection of participating practicing physicians is a joint effort of physician leaders and the relevant IHCDS executive, and/or (where applicable) board or management committee.

Practicing physicians selected to participate with management on these occasions will have relevant clinical training and experience, a reputation for objectivity and fairness, good analytical skills, and good communication skills.

Definition of Relevant Authority

Individuals and groups making decisions affecting the delivery of medical services include:

- The system board.
- The system CEO.
- The board of any system component (if applicable, such as if a hospital or medical center board retains decision-making authority in some areas).
- The CEO, chief operating officer, or vice president in charge of any system component.
- The vice president for medical affairs of the system.
- The vice president for medical affairs or medical director of system components (such as hospital or medical center, mental health services, ambulatory care services, etc.).

Definition of Decisions Affecting the Delivery of Medical Care Services

Decisions affecting delivery of medical care services include but are not necessarily limited to:

1. Planning, construction, and/or renovation of patient care service areas.

2. Mergers with or acquisitions of other health care service institutions/organizations in the served area.

3. New alliances with physicians in the area served by the system.

4. Staffing for various patient care areas, including nurses and other patient care personnel, such as technicians and therapists.

5. Selection of the staff of practicing physicians, including primary care physicians and the cadre of specialists and subspecialists on whom practicing physicians are dependent for clinical consultation in a variety of circumstances.

6. Selection of a clinical support services group, such as pathology or radiology/imaging services.

7. Decision about what services shall be provided by the various components of the integrated health care delivery system.

8. Selection of senior executives, as relevant to the activities of practicing physicians.

9. Selection of members of the board of directors of the system and of any system component.

10. Funding of education and training programs for clinical personnel, including nurses, technicians, and therapists.

11. Establishment of reserve funds for capital improvements and contingencies.

Participation Mechanisms

Specific mechanisms might include, but are not necessarily limited to:

- Practicing physicians with relevant clinical training and experience on relevant management committees and executive work groups.

- Physician leaders as full members of relevant board and executive committees.

- Preparation of fact analyses, position papers, and/or specific recommendations by relevant physician leaders, at the request of the relevant board or management committee or work group.

Participation of practicing physicians (through implementation of this policy) is reflected in written proceedings, such as minutes and reports, of relevant board and management committees and work groups.

Approved _____

Date _____

*Thompson, R. *So You've Been Integrated, Now What? Opportunities for Physicians Practicing in Managed Care Settings.* Tampa, Fla.: American College of Physician Executives, 1996, pp. 72-3.

Figure 2. An Old Sample Position Description for a Corporate VPMA

May 10, 1993

Position

Corporate/System Vice President for Medical Affairs (VPMA)

Position Overview

The system's corporate vice president for medical affairs is the primary advocate ensuring that considerations of dependable clinical performance are included in executive/management decisions at the corporate and institution level.

The corporate VPMA develops, describes, and wins support for necessary and desirable activities ranging from strategic planning, through education/development of the medical staff and medical staff leaders, to specifics of assessing physician performance through credentialing and recredentialing. In addition, this individual is involved in physician recruitment and retention, helping physicians view the system and its component locations as preferred practice opportunities.

Selected by:

The corporate CEO, with advice and consent of the system's board of directors and with input from the system's medical advisory committee and from the CEO and medical executive committee of each system component location.

Reports to:

The system CEO

Subordinate Reporting Relationships

Option 1: This is a staff resource position; no one reports to the VPMA.

Option 2: This is a line position; some combination of the following report to the VPMA:

- Corporate Director of QI/PA

- Corporate Director of Risk Management

- Corporate Director of Physician Recruitment and Retention

- VPMA (Medical Director) of each system location (if there is one)

Relates to:

The system/corporate VPMA interacts with many individuals and groups, including, but not necessarily limited to:

- The system's board of directors.

- The system's medical advisory committee.

- The system's corporate office staff, as relevant and indicated.

- CEO (COO?) of each system location.

- Elected medical staff leaders (officers and clinical department chairs, committee chairs and members) at each system location.

- Others, such as nursing leaders, both corporate and local, as relevant and indicated.

Qualifications

The system's VPMA must have an MD or a DO degree. Beyond that, personal leadership qualities of the individual are probably more important than further formal training (such as an MBA).

Past experience in clinical practice is desirable, although this position does not include the opportunity for clinical practice. (Because the individual will not be practicing, licensure is optional.) Where clinical knowledge and judgment are required, this individual's work will consist of mobilizing current clinical expertise of physicians comprising the medical staffs of system locations, not providing specific clinical expertise him- or herself.

The position requires an individual willing to travel, spending time as needed on location in system institutions, and to work irregular hours as may be made necessary by such tasks as attending evening meetings.

The corporate VPMA should have good communications skills, both oral and written. He or she should be conversant with and experienced in applying conflict resolution skills.

Specific Tasks

Note: The initial job description should not be rigid. Rather, it should sketch objectives and tasks in broad strokes. The individual chosen to fill the position should work with both corporate and local leaders to fill in further details as the position is implemented.

The work of the system's VPMA includes, but is not necessarily limited to:

1. Serve as liaison between the systemwide medical advisory committee and the system's board of directors.

2. Working with local medical staff leaders, serve as liaison between:

    - The MAC and practitioners at system locations.

    - Corporate office staff and physician leaders and frontline practitioners at System locations.

3. Help local medical staff leaders communicate effectively with the board and the executive staff and with frontline clinicians at their own locations.

4. Staff the corporate medical advisory committee.

5. With the system's medical advisory committee, create consistency (not "standardization," just consistency) in relevant rules, policies, procedures, bylaws, and methods in system institutions.

    Example: Without insisting on "corporate model" medical staff bylaws, the corporate VPMA and the medical advisory committee should suggest certain consistent features of the credentialing process at each system location.

6. Assist with selecting and implementing the most advantageous (to the system, its component parts, and its physicians) structures for relating each physician to the system, given prevalent market factors in a given area.

Example: Physician-Hospital Organizations (PHOs)

7. Assist system's locations in retaining accreditation by the Joint Commission on Accreditation of Healthcare Organizations in the medical staff/board, "leadership," and "quality improvement/performance assessment" areas.

8. Help relevant individuals and groups within the system and its locations identify the need for, and implement, needed health care services in communities served by the system.

9. Help both corporate and local leaders (medical, executive/management, and governing body leaders) develop mutually beneficial cooperative efforts with other health care centers in geographical areas served by the system and its component parts.

10. Assist, as requested, with efforts to recruit and retain physicians in communities served by the system, such as:

    • Assist physicians, as appropriate and requested, with office practice management, data processing systems, and orientation and continuing education of office staff.

    • Assist in establishing services that can be offered to the system's physicians, such as assistance in negotiating contracts with managed care groups, etc.

11. Assist in establishing an orientation program for new physician staff members.

12. On a regular basis, meet with, advise, and receive input from the CEO group (the CEO of the system and the CEO of each system location) about physician issues, interests, and concerns.

13. At each location, assist in establishing positive relationships between the medical staff and nursing service.

14. Help design and implement innovations, such as acceptance of using financial information in assessment of physician performance.

15. Coach individual physicians on how best to make interests and concerns heard by executive staffs and boards at both the local and the corporate levels.

16. Be available, as relevant and indicated, to facilitate the resolution of conflicts (be a "trouble-shooter").

17. Supervise development and implementation of a systematic schedule of continuing medical education opportunities at each system location.

18. If appropriate, pursue the possibility of appropriate linkages with accredited medical schools, to promote medical teaching in the system's locations.

Chapter 10

Ten 1991 Predictions Revisited, Plus One

In the 1980s, dubbed by some "The Greed Decade," over-promising in advertising and exploitive profit-taking were prevalent in the health care business. This is not surprising, because exploitation of the public and of employees was our national business ethic at that time. "Who says life has to be fair?" was our watchword. On the last episode of the TV drama, Dallas, ruthless business tycoon J. R. Ewing was asked, "J.R., what's your secret to being such a successful businessman?" "Secret?" answered J.R. "There's no secret. Once you give up integrity, everything else is a piece a cake."

The ten "safe" predictions in the first edition of this book (1991)[1] were based on the hope that health care executives and physicians were on the verge of rediscovering that total value is the proven key to sustaining a profit-making business.

Total Value = Reasonable Cost *plus* Dependable Services

> *When the goal is profit, the result is often disappointment. But when the goal is delivering dependable goods and services, the result is usually profit.*

This was not just wishful thinking, because in 1991 the popularity of then-"new" continuous quality improvement (CQI) principles made this assumption reasonable. The 14 CQI principles, made famous by Dr. W. Edwards Deming,[2] include "(#1) Create constancy of purpose" because "the purpose of business rather than making money is to stay in business and provide jobs," and "(#4) End the practice of awarding business on price tag alone." Furthermore, when Dr. Deming advised "(#9) Break down barriers between staff areas," I'm sure he did not have the unique executive/physician relationship in mind, but he might as well have.

But today, CQI exists in name only in many managed care organizations, while the real guiding paradigm is no different than in the 1980s. That is, in spite of eloquent statements of mission and purpose, the real operational guideline remains, "Get the money, keep the money, and do not let calls for 'quality' deter you from your quest. After all, who says life has to be fair?" This paradigm reflects instant gratification, not the long range goal of "stay in business."

So, in the health care business, we find that the old Chinese proverb is still relevant: "If we do not change our direction, we are very likely to end up exactly where we are headed."

In that light, here are the ten 1991 predictions about the executive/physician relationship, updated to reflect both events of the 1990s and anticipation of assumptions and actions of the executive/physician leadership team in the immediate future. Plus, an eleventh prediction has been added to the list.

1. *Mutual trust will increase.* In the first edition, I explained that this was not a suggestion that "executives and physicians would suddenly, magically, see only the best in each other." Rather, I suggested that "this relationship, like many others, will be helped by rediscovery of basic values that once made the United States a leader nation."

    Well, I didn't say when. I stand by this prediction. Again, this is not just wishful thinking. Part of the 1991 prediction was, "Management gurus will laud mutual benefits of cooperative effort." This is just now beginning to happen.[3-5]

2. *Physician input to governing body and executive decisions will be more effective.* This is true. In 1991, many physicians still tended to use opportunities to provide input as forums to deliver demands. But today, all but the most traditionally thinking physicians understand how organizations work and how to influence senior management decisions.[6] ACPE's courses, seminars, and publications deserve a great deal of credit for this development. So do pioneer VPMAs in many health care settings.

3. *Physicians will choose to be part of winning health care organizations.* True. After a phase in which some physician groups try to be "providers" in the total organizational sense, the health care system will settle into what it must eventually be. That is, we will have a national network of health care professionals providing clinical services in organizations run in a business-like manner by individuals with executive training.

    Part of this 1991 prediction was that "frantic attempts to buy a physician's loyalty will not be pursued." At least we are out of the era in which some executives foolishly believed that loyalty of a physician or of a physician's patients can be bought. Loyalty of a sought-after physician has to be earned by providing dependable nursing staff and by making only promises that can and will be kept in a timely manner. Plus, of course, loyalty can be demanded by contract.

    And the 1991 prediction characterized a "winning health care organization" as one in which "the stranglehold of legalisms and bureaucracy will be broken by proactive thinking." By that definition, winning organizations are, at this writing, few and far between. Today, the biggest buzzword in health care is "compliance."

But, again, I didn't say when. I'll stand by this prediction. It is now possible, for example, to place a cover sheet on some documents related to medical staff organizational functions that clarifies that "this particular document does not require legal review!"[7]

Unfortunately, it's necessary to revise this prediction to point out that total involvement in "compliance" contributes to our ethical immaturity, which could turn out to be the fatal flaw in a managed care organization (see Chapter 6).

4. *Health care organizations will choose sought-after practitioners.* "As it was in the beginning, it is now and ever shall be." There has been no change in the definition of "sought-after physician" since 1991, and it is unlikely that there ever will be much change in this definition. A sought-after physician is one with the following characteristics and behavior:

- Carefully applies updated clinical knowledge and skills to each patient.

- Is cooperative and pleasant with fellow practitioners, health care center personnel, patients, and family members.

- Appreciates contributions of others to the care of patients for whom he or she is responsible.

- Dependably fulfills the obligations of the medical profession, including ready accessibility (or provision for readily accessible coverage) in the event of an emergency.

- Completes patient records (manual or electronic) accurately, legibly, and in a timely manner.

- Practices efficiently. That is, keeps concern for desirable patient care results the number one priority, but also considers the expense of ordered tests, treatments, and health care services.

5. *Students in health care management degree programs will be taught how to work with physicians, nurses, and other health care professionals.* Forget it. It looks like this is never going to happen.

> *I had experience working with (hospital management) students...who never had exposure to a nurse or a doctor. The one opportunity they had to understand what a doctor or a nurse does (their training) had been blown. They need to understand what makes a nurse and a doctor work, what are their value judgments, and how to get them to be a part of the team.*—H. Robert Cathcart, President and CEO, Pennsylvania Hospital, Philadelphia.

Today, with few exceptions, entering health care executives are still left to learn "what makes doctors (and nurses) work" from difficult experiences and books like this one.

6.   *More chief executive officers will be physicians and nurses with executive training and experience.* In 1991, the chief financial officer had the inside track to replace a moving or retiring CEO. Today, the edge may belong to an experienced VPMA. That's because the CFO's view of the organization is usually very narrow, while VPMAs usually have a broader perspective. And the CEO who was formerly a VPMA can always hire and depend on a good CFO.

7.   *Successful physicians will broaden their notion of patient care.* True. Traditionally thinking physicians who define clinical care only as "me and my patient!" now find themselves on the outside looking in.

8.   *Health care organizations will temper competitive practices with social concerns.* Dead wrong, so far. Chapter 6 of this second edition contains a stronger appeal for achieving personal and organizational success through ethically mature approaches to the health care business.

9.   *As patient care protocols evolve, fewer physicians will be needed.* Actually, I should have said fewer specialists and subspecialists and more primary care practitioners. But at all three levels of care, fewer physicians may now be needed as health care services increasingly integrate and as clinical guidelines become the norm in guiding some aspects of care.

In addition, enter independent clinical practitioners (ICPs) of various disciplines. More and more, instead of "I'm Doctor Welby's patient," one hears, "I'm in the MediBest Health Care Plan." And MediBest leaders have an intense interest in expanding credentialing and privileging to include a variety of ICPs. The interest, of course, is the hope that these "allied health professionals" will work cheaper. But effective professional organizations representing these ICPs are making it quite clear that this isn't going to happen. The value of "physician extenders" is the (real or perceived) increased dependability of health care services. For example, in some clinical settings the interpersonal skills of allied professionals are better than those of many physicians. Another example is that a qualified nurse practitioner or a clinical technician now often has more in-depth knowledge of a specialized or subspecialized field than the average physician.

10.   *At the medical center of 2001, the nature of the "organized medical staff" (in hospitals) will have changed.* True. In the 1990s, we have gone through an era of "reengineering" the *structure* of the organized medical staff in U.S. hospitals. Today, we are just beginning the era of reengineering *functional methods* by which tasks such as cre-

dentialing and privileging are accomplished.[7]

The prediction that "the medical executive function will reside in a VPMA working with a small physician cabinet, rather than in a large medical executive committee" is not yet true, but we're moving in that direction.

Finally, one new prediction:

11. *By the end of the second decade of the new millennium, providers and medical professionals will have recaptured health care from government interference and insurance company exploitive profit-taking.* This will happen because the public will demand that it happen as soon as it becomes clear that so many people's health care dollars are not being spent to deliver health care. That is, the existing system is characterized more by legal, financial, and political maneuvering and by draining money out of the system than by building up reserves for training, education, research, contingencies, and replacement costs. Ideally, the public demand will come soon enough to stave off the next predictable phase of the current implementation of "managed care," which is a rash of hospital and health care organization bankruptcies.

The central players in this return of sanity to the health care field will be the powerful executive/physician shared leadership teams around the country who eschew infighting and bickering and pursue cooperative efforts that include developing a shared ethic and using it as an operational guideline.

In this new age, some providers and professionals will still choose to cut out "third-party" insurance companies and perform the insurance function themselves. This financing model will be far superior to the current financing model of health care. That's because, after reasonable profit-taking (or staying within budget, including handsome remuneration for physicians and executives, if the financing model is by then a single-payer model), the physician/executive leadership team will use a larger number of people's health care dollars to pay for providing dependable health care services.

Note that this prediction will not come true unless the physician/executive leadership team continues to evolve and comes forward boldly to lead a provider/professional/public coalition that must negotiate from strength with the politician/insurer complex.[8]

Discussion Points

Here are some factors that will greatly affect the evolution of the executive/physician shared leadership team. Discuss your own predictions about each one of these factors.

1. Distrust in the physician/executive relationship is in part a reflection of lack of trust

as a national malaise. Do you believe there will be a restoration of public trust in government and "big business?" Why or why not? Wouldn't restoration of trust first require a return to integrity (honesty) in business and government? If so, are there any current factors that could drive such a rediscovery of the economic value of integrity? If so, what are they?

2. Do you agree that many physicians today provide reasonable and articulate suggestions to the executive/management staff? Or do physicians still just make demands on management and expect their "authority as physicians" to force those demands to be met?

3. Will bitter battles for "covered lives" continue? Or will groups of institutional providers, primary care physicians, and clinical specialists and subspecialists learn to participate together in value-added ventures?

4. Will current stirrings of a positive, professional approach to matters such as credentialing physicians and using performance information survive? Or will they be buried under an avalanche of legalistic debris created by lawyers for health care organizations and physicians?

5. Look again at the definition of a "sought-after practitioner" in Prediction #4 and the accompanying statement that "it is unlikely that there ever will be much change in this definition." Do you agree or disagree?

6. Will basic training of health care managers and executives begin to include education about what makes doctors and nurses tick?

7. Will some remnants of health care as a critical public service be retained in the next phases of managed care? Or is Bud Selig right; "Baseball is just a business," and so is health care?

8. Will boards tend to select more CEOs from the available pool of physician executives?

9. Will the evolution of clinical practice guidelines and critical clinical pathways eventually make the phenomenon of clinical decision making unnecessary and thus take away the physician's primary source of organizational power?

10. In which direction will the position of VPMA develop? Toward being an extension of the financial goals of the organization? Toward being responsible for issues once dealt with as well as possible by a volunteer "chief of staff" and a "medical staff coordinator?" In both directions? Is this really two positions? Or is some alternative other than the above likely?

11. What predictions of your own would you add to the list of predictions in this chapter?

References

1. Thompson, R. *Keys to Winning Physician Support*, First Edition. Tampa, Fla.: American College of Physician Executives, 1991, p. 79.

2. Walton, M. *The Deming Management Method*. New York, N.Y., Perigree, 1986.

3. Coile, R. *The Five Stages of Managed Care: Strategies for Providers, HMO's and Suppliers*. Chicago, Ill.: Health Administration Press, 1997.

4. Dodge, D. "Competition Is Dead: Long Live Competition!" *InnerViews* Nov.-Dec. 1996, p. 2.

5. Moore, J. *The Death of Competition: Leadership and Strategy in the Age of Business Ecosystems*. New York, N.Y.: HarperBusiness, 1996.

6. Thompson, Richard E. "How to Exercise Power When You Have Limited Authority." *Family Practice Management* 5(1):82-3, Jan. 1998.

7. *Medical Staff Portfolio*, Second Edition. Dunedin, Fla.: Thompson, Mohr and Associates, Inc., 1996.

8. Thompson, R. "Health Care Reform: Believe It or Not, the Ball Is Back in Our Court." *Physician Executive* 20(12):9-13, Dec. 1994.

Appendix
Cases for Discussion

In a reflective setting, such as a leadership retreat with a skilled moderator either from within your organization or from the outside, discuss one or more of these true-to-life scenarios.

Discuss cases that are not similar to current issues in your organization. The purpose of this exercise is not to solve current problems. It is to practice discussing sensitive topics as objectively as possible, avoiding emotional baggage related to past events, personalities, local political alliances, and not-so-hidden agendas.

An unavoidable serendipity of this exercise will be further understanding of the concept of ethical maturity (see Chapter 6) and of its usefulness and value in the business world.

The Case of the "Managed Care" Conflict in a Lovely Resort Location

A nationwide health care system convened its executives, senior managers, and key local physician leaders in a nice resort location for a two-day brainstorming session right before the planning retreat of the board of directors. The stated purpose was to obtain physician input for use by the board in planning further evolution of this already successful organization.

I. Costa Bigbux, MD, MBA, a circuit-riding facilitator well known to the management team but not to physician members of the group, was engaged to moderate both the two-day brainstorming session and the board's planning retreat.

On the first day of the retreat, in spite of Costa's best efforts, discussions bogged down because of total disagreement about whether "managed care" is good or bad and whether or not it is really here to stay.

Physicians in the group berated management for "ruining the patient-physician relationship," for pushing too-absolute adherence to practice guidelines, and for cutting costs in ways that showed they "don't understand patient care."

Members of the management team countered by suggesting that one doesn't have to be a doctor to know what's best for patients. Some told of their personal experiences as patients in the hospital and insisted they received excellent care. The CFO advised the doctors to realize a basic truth: "No margin, no medicine."

On the second day of the retreat, taking a suggestion made by people seated at his table at the previous night's banquet, Costa suggested that the group seemed to be using the term "managed care" to mean more than one thing. He suggested that careful definition of terms might help members of the group avoid arguing when they do not really disagree, which should allow productive interaction to occur.

To start the discussion, Costa offered the following "first-draft definitions" and asked the group to suggest how these definitions should be modified in order to be acceptable:

Managed Care is sometimes used to refer to the current U.S. health care policy of "managed competition," unique in the world because the primary goal is maximizing investor profit.

Managed Care is also used to mean management of the individual patient or client or resident using practice guidelines.

Managed Care Organization (MCO) means an entity that exists only on paper. The purpose of an MCO is to take advantage of current national and state health care policy that encourages profit-taking with one hand while ratcheting down revenues to providers with the other.

Managed Competition refers to current U.S. health care policy. Competition is "managed" by a complex set of federal and state laws and regulations.

IDS means Integrated Delivery System. An IDS is simply an integrated network of health care professionals and supporting managers that provides a convenient and efficient opportunity for people in need of any health care service to receive it from the same provider. The term IDS is not synonymous with managed care organization and does not imply any specific funding mechanism.

Costa's suggestion was unanimously rejected by the group. The physician members of the group said that they did not give up their weekend just to play silly word games. Members of the management team said that, meaning no disrespect to either him or his dinner companions, this was really not what they had come to discuss. They told him they preferred to "skip the philosophy" and take up and make decisions about several specific issues.

The result was a second day of bickering and bogged-down, circular discussions, during which many members of the group left early so they could enjoy the resort with their families.

The next week, back home, everyone agreed that the weekend had been a dismal failure except for the family fun, some great food and acceptable wine, and a hole-in-one by B. Mia Caddy, the Director of Nursing.

Discussion Starters

1. Could any advance preparations have avoided the counterproductive first day? Selection of participants? Orientation of physician participants, who may not be experienced in "the group process?" Was Costa the right choice of retreat facilitator/resource? If so, why? If not, why not? Should physician participants participate in selecting the "outside resource" for such a retreat? Should the purpose have been more clearly thought through and stated ahead of time...something more specific than "to obtain physician input?"

2. How could anyone but a doctor know what is best for patients?

3. Can the CEO know how well "ordinary patients" are cared for by extrapolating from his or her own experience as a hospitalized patient?

4. Is "No margin, no medicine" or "No margin, no mission" ever used by anyone as an excuse for exploitive profit-taking?

5. Do physicians ever use an expressed concern for "quality" to pursue their own goals?

6. In your discussions with each other, are you using the term "managed care" to mean more than one thing? If so, could this be contributing to misunderstandings and perceived disagreements? If you take the time to carefully define the various uses of the term "managed care," should you expect that all disagreements about whether managed care is good or bad will dissolve?

7. What changes would you make in Costa's "first draft definitions?" Would you add any terms? Subract any? Would you reword any of Costa's definitions? How?

The Case of the Pampered Practitioner

Ima Jeenyus, MD, a physician with a subspecialty in a field that is a large revenue-producer for hospitals, had long been a golfing buddy of Sam Sentinel, President of the First National Bank and Chairman of the MMC (Merged Medical Center) board. Three months ago, on the eleventh tee, Ima suggested to Sam that the hospital could make a lot of money by "going together" with him to offer a new risky surgical procedure that Ima had just learned but in which he claimed proficiency. "See one, do one, teach one, you know," joked Ima, shanking his drive into the trees.

When Sam told other board members and the CEO of this opportunity, they were thrilled and voted to implement the idea immediately.

Medical staff president R.U. Sure, MD and credentials coordinator Dewey Needyu registered objections. "Dr. Jeenyus' technical skills are beyond question," they agreed, but they pointed out that "the board has not yet responded to our concerns about seven instances of questionable surgical judgment in his practice."

The board thanked R.U. and Dewey for their input and asked that the formality of processing Ima's application for this additional "clinical privilege" be expedited.

Needed instruments and equipment were obtained, Ima was given a high priority on the operating suite schedule, temporary privileges to perform the new procedure were granted, and the marketing department ran a full-page ad in the local newspaper, featuring an action shot of Ima in a surgical scrubsuit.

At the time of the next board meeting, when Ima's formal credentials application was ready for action by the Board, there had been no mishaps related to technical aspects of the procedure. However...

There had already been one instance in which Ima was so eager to practice his new craft that, without consulting the patient's referring physician, he discontinued a patient's anticoagulant drug for 48 hours prior to scheduled surgery so that he could proceed with his (possibly unnecessary) operation without fear of excessive bleeding. The operation was a success, and the patient was placed back on his regular medications including the anticoagulant drug and was discharged home.

The physician analyst who monitors data and daily observations reflecting physician performance suggested that Ima and the hospital, not to mention Ima's patient, had dodged a bullet. She suggested that Ima's privilege to perform the new procedure be suspended until this instance and the previous seven instances of questionable clinical judgment could be discussed with Ima and resolved.

Discussion Starters

1. Should the board chair discuss hospital business with a doctor on the golf course? Without the CEO present? Is there a more appropriate way for Dr. Jeenyus to make his proposal? If so, why would Dr. Jeenyus think he should make his proposal during a round of golf with the board chair?

2. Should a CEO and board consider any factors other than projected revenues when adding a physician to the medical staff or adding a new clinical service to the managed care organization's "product line?"

3. How do you suppose Dr. Sure and Dr. Needyu learned that this deal was in the works?

4. If Dr. Sure and Dr. Needyu are going to obstruct potentially profitable business ventures in this way, why not replace them?

5. Did Dr. Sure and Dr. Needyu have a point? Did they express their objection in a reasonable and articulate manner?

6. Is this board practicing shared leadership?

7. What might be some of the immediate and long-term results or consequences of this scenario, depending on what happens next?

8. What should the CEO have done, if anything, and at what point?

9. Because the patient "did well," was it overzealous for the physician analyst to suggest that this "near miss" be called to Ima's attention?

10. Are your answers reflective of your organization's ethics committee's policy on patient rights and ethics?

The Case of the .38 Special

An oncologist diagnosed a child as having a far-advanced, untreatable malignant tumor; that is, an untreatable cancer. (Pediatrics is not all "well child care.") The pediatric oncologist talked to the child's pediatrician regarding next steps. Among other things, they decided to hold a same-day conference with the parents to break this devastating news. They asked the chaplain member of the hospital's ethics committee to attend this conference with the parents to offer immediate support and to become acquainted with the clinical nature of this case in the event the ethics committee's guidance might be needed at some point in the dying child's clinical course. The chaplain had a previous engagement and could not come.

That afternoon, the pediatrician and oncologist informed the parents that their daughter had an untreatable, fatal disease and would soon die. The mother pulled a .38-special revolver from her purse, brandished it at the two doctors, and said, "If my daughter dies, you die." The parents then left the room (after the mother had put the gun back in her purse), leaving the two frightened physicians sitting pale, paralyzed, speechless, and in a quandary.

Discussion Starters

1. Should the physicians report this incident? If so, to whom?

2. Should this incident be documented? If so, how?

3. Should the police be notified?

4. Was the chaplain's response appropriate? If not, what should he have done?

5. In your hospital, where would the doctors and the parents have held this sensitive conference? That is, are private rooms set aside for this purpose, out of the traffic pattern and ensured to be free of interruption?

6. In your organization, is there a written policy to be followed in such an instance that answers those questions? If so, did physician leaders participate in developing this policy?

7. If there is a written policy, was it FFF'ed (finished, filed, and forgotten), or are the hospital's physicians oriented to this policy and reminded of it from time to time? If so, how much of the responsibility for this communication to frontline clinicians belongs to key medical staff leaders, such as chairs or directors of clinical departments or of major clinical services?

8. Are you practicing shared leadership in this area?

The Case of the Lost Leader

Dr. Meaghan Kairs has been a very valuable physician leader for several years. But now she is disappointed and frustrated.

The medical executive leadership in her hospital (which is unbelievably complicated, consisting of the short-term medical staff president and permanent VPMA, plus an 11-member medical executive committee, plus someone called the CEO) asked Meaghan to coordinate "medical staff performance improvement" activities. The tasks include being a physician advisor to the performance improvement office, monitoring data and daily observations reflecting physician performance.

Meaghan was told that the position would not require much time, because it was just something that had been set up in response to some requirements by the Joint Commission. But Meaghan didn't see it that way. For one thing, Meaghan had observed, during the course of her hospital practice, some opportunities for improving clinical systems that she was eager to help implement. In addition, she was excited about the potential opportunity to smooth out peaks and valleys in the organizational skills of elected leaders. That is, she had noted that some department chairs had good organizational skills and some didn't. She felt that she could help department chairs perform their duties related to maintaining dependable clinical performance in the hospital.

In addition, she felt she could demonstrate her belief that "confronting" physicians about the need to change clinical practice habits need not mean pulling the bylaws on them. Rather, Meaghan was sure that most physicians would respond to a professional appeal that was carefully prepared, correctly presented, and backed up by current articles in the medical "literature." She was eager to help "coach" clinical department chairs and their designees who are responsible for talking with physicians to motivate improved performance.

After eight months, Meaghan is quite pleased with her visible contributions to patient care systems, working with nursing and other clinical departments. In addition to the satisfaction of improving patient care, Meaghan's contributions are being acknowledged by nursing leadership and the executive staff.

In addition, Meaghan feels great professional satisfaction because of the fact that three clinical department chairs have welcomed her help and have told her she has really helped them understand the duties of a department chair.

But Meaghan is frustrated that several physician performance issues discovered through routine data-gathering and daily observations (as opposed to witch-hunt type "studies" of an individual physician's practice) are still listed as "unresolved." Meaghan believes in reasonable clinical controversy. She's not trying to get people to practice her way. These are issues that endanger patients, colleagues, and/or hospital personnel.

The problem is lack of action by a few clinical department chairs. Rather than welcoming Meaghan's help, they seem to view it as interference with their prerogatives. They will neither take the bull by the horns nor lend Meaghan their authority. All they are willing to do is call a departmental committee meeting and discuss the issues that Meaghan refers to them. Meaghan has indicated her willingness to attend these meetings to try to be helpful, but she has not been invited to do so. Invariably, the meetings end with a voted decision that Meaghan's interpretation of relevant information is incorrect and that the department concludes that "care was appropriate."

Meaghan figures that, even though she's made some positive contributions, if these most important issues can't be addressed, her position is ineffective and she is basically wasting her time.

So Meaghan is resigning. Her resignation letter, which the medical staff president promises to present to the medical executive committee, concludes with announcing her decision to decline any further offers to assume a position of medical staff leadership.

Discussion Starters

1. What would you do, if anything, to simplify the "medical executive" function in this hospital (component of an integrated delivery system)?

2. Is Meagan overzealous? That is, why is she so concerned that department chairs act? Could this inaction cause any undesirable consequences for the hospital? For the hospital's physicians? For the integrated delivery system or managed care organization of which this hospital is a part? (Think about your answer in terms of public image, marketing success, potential legal problems, and the board's obligation to ensure good patient care results).

3. Why won't the reluctant department chairs act?

4. Should the medical staff president try to talk Meaghan out of resigning?

5. Is it good or bad that Meaghan has held positions of responsible leadership on the medical staff for so long? Shouldn't these responsibilities be "passed around?"

6. What should the VPMA's role, if any, be in this scenario?

7. What should the CEO's role, if any, be in this scenario?

8. What should the board's role, if any, be in this scenario?

The Case of the Military Mission

At the annual meeting of the executive staff, board, and physician leaders of a successful integrated delivery network, Day One opened with a prayer and devotional by Sister Withit, Director of Missions. Then the morning session was spent discussing, revising, and eventually approving a truly eloquent and moving statement about caring, compassion, and social responsibility.

During long-range planning discussions on Day Two, Dr. Newtoo Thisgame, a physician leader from one of the system's smallest hospitals, proposed that, in light of yesterday's pledge to consider the needs of the community, it might be time to consider burying the hatchet with the cross-town hospital in his community (owned by a different system). He pointed out that, if a cooperative working relationship were developed between the two hospitals, it should be possible to avoid expensive duplication of health care services in the community.

A few doctors applauded. The executives and managers in the group audibly gasped. The vice president of marketing jeeringly asked, "Doctor, do you really think that General Patton discussed his battle plans with the Nazis?"

Discussion Starters

1. Was Day One of this retreat valuable? Or should the group have "gotten right down to business?"

2. What is the purpose of creating a "shared ethic" statement with physician leader participation? Is there any value beyond meeting external requirements for such statements?

3. Was Dr. Thisgame out of order?

4. Is there any way to avoid "group surprises" such as Dr. Thisgame's? What steps would you take in planning and conducting such a retreat to offer group members an opportunity to present new ideas?

5.   Why are physician leaders more likely to applaud cooperative community efforts while business managers and executives are more likely either to emphasize "competition" or to fear such joint efforts because of antitrust issues?

6.   Did the vice president of marketing make his point effectively? Is it okay that the CEO handles working with physicians, leaving other members of the executive team free of any concern for working well with physicians?

7.   What, if anything, would you do to further the development of shared leadership with physicians in this system?

The Case of the Emergency Call Coverage Impasse

The medical staff bylaws revision and organizational restructuring project was almost finished, and in record time at that. At the beginning, Dr. I. Ben Trubble had urged that, in contrast with the process for previous bylaws projects, the drafting committee not get stuck on debating such issues as whether the list of officers should be "president and president-elect" or "chief of staff and vice chief."

Expressing the view of several physicians on the project committee, Dr. Trubble pointed out that the project should be completed post-haste so that physicians could spend their time on new issues related to the recently developed physician/hospital organization and the securing of managed care contracts.

In spite of that view, the project bogged down because of an impasse at the point of "emergency services backup coverage." Some physicians pointed out that, once upon a time, emergency department coverage was desirable as a source of new patients but now, especially with some "managed care physicians" balking at being included on the back-up call schedule, coverage and follow-up responsibilities for "assigned patients" was becoming a burden, especially for a few physicians.

After several attempts to draft compromise language, all of which were rejected for some good reason or another, Dr. N.O. Vater suggested a totally new approach. "Who is it," he asked rhetorically, "that wants the emergency department covered? The answer," he continued, "is the hospital executive staff and board, because in our state a hospital cannot keep its license unless emergency services are provided on a round-the-clock, seven-days-a-week basis." Therefore, Dr. Vater wondered, why not finish the bylaws project with only a general reference to emergency department coverage and have a group of executives and physicians get together to identify some doctors who would be willing to "cover the emergency department" if paid to do so and indemnified, perhaps from a joint fund established by a board appropriation and medical staff dues assessment?

Some physicians were interested in the idea, but several balked at the notion of having to pay extra dues. The CEO told the group that he had never heard of such an arrangement and that there was no money in the budget for it anyway, so it would be best for the group to just keep trying to solve the problem through mandating emergency department coverage in the medical staff bylaws.

Discussion Starters

1. Do some doctors on medical staff bylaws committees really still get bogged down discussing such issues as "Chief or President" vs. "Chief-Elect or President-Elect?"

2. How important is the traditional organized medical staff today, compared to the importance of timely participation in shared leadership by committed and skilled physician leaders?

3. Dr. Ben Trubble, once an obstructionist who opposed practically any proposed bylaws change, is now for getting on with completing the bylaws revision project and dealing with other issues. What do you suppose caused this turnaround in attitude?

4. "Emergency services backup coverage" by physicians is a common problem. Why is that, do you suppose?

5. Is there any merit in Dr. N.O. Vater's suggestion?

6. Whether there is or not, could or should the CEO have proceeded any differently than to reject Dr. Vater's suggestion without discussion?

7. Is a medical staff bylaws revision the best way to resolve today's issues related to physician responsibilities to the organization, the organization's responsibility to physicians, and the responsibility of both the organization and its physicians to people needing and using health care services?

8. Should Dr. Trubble be invited to share in organizational leadership? Or does his past history of being an obstructionist rob him of that opportunity?

9. Is shared leadership being practiced in this hospital? If so, how? If not, why not?

10. In your organization, are there any issues that have caused impasses in the past that might be better resolved through innovative new approaches involving shared leadership? If so, what are one or two examples?